Dr. W. R.

600 MCQs in Anaesthe

600 MCQs in Anaesthesia: Clinical Practice

P. J. Simpson
MD FFARCS
Consultant Anaesthetist,
Frenchay Hospital, Bristol;
Senior Clinical Lecturer,
University of Bristol, UK

N. W. Goodman
MA DPhil BM BCh FFARCS
Lecturer in Anaesthesia,
University of Bristol, UK

Churchill Livingstone
EDINBURGH LONDON MELBOURNE AND NEW YORK 1987

CHURCHILL LIVINGSTONE
Medical Division of Longman Group UK Limited

Distributed in the United States of America by Churchill Livingstone Inc., 1560 Broadway, New York, N.Y. 10036, and by associated companies, branches and representatives throughout the world.

First published 1987

ISBN 0-443-03155-X

British Library Cataloguing in Publication Data
Simpson, Peter J.
600 MCQs in anaesthesia: clinical practice.
1. Anesthesia — Problems, exercises, etc.
I. Title II. Goodman, N. W.
617'.96'076 RD82.3

Library of Congress Cataloging in Publication Data
Simpson, Peter J.
600 MCQs in anaesthesia. Clinical practice.

Companion volume to: 600 MCQs in anaesthesia. Basic sciences.
Includes index.
1. Anesthesiology — Examinations, questions, etc.
I. Goodman, N. W. II. Title. III. Title: Six hundred MCQs in anaesthesia. [DNLM: 1. Anesthesiology — examination questions. WO 218 S613za]
RD82.3.S476 1986 617'.96'076 86-14728

Produced by Longman Singapore Publishers (Pte) Limited
Printed in Singapore

Preface

This book aims to provide examination practice at Multiple Choice Questions on Clinical Practice for the diploma of the FFARCS. The questions are arranged in mock papers of 60 MCQs to allow candidates to time themselves answering questions on a range of topics likely to be encountered in the written and oral section of Parts I and III of the examination. It will help with the need to get a 'feel' for MCQ technique before turning to the 'real thing' in the examination hall.

Unlike those books of MCQs arranged under topic headings, candidates will have to be adaptable, not only to changing topic from question to question, but also to the degree of difficulty — and, as is bound to happen in the actual examination, candidates will find that there are some questions which they cannot answer.

As with the companion volume of questions on the Basic Sciences, the compilation of the papers was eased by the powerful word-processing facilities of a DEC PDP-11 computer; and again we must acknowledge the help of colleagues and candidates past and present in the Nuffield Department of Anaesthetics, Oxford, and in the three Teaching Hospitals in Bristol: Southmead, Frenchay and Bristol Royal Infirmary.

Bristol,
1987

P. J. S.
N. W. G.

Introduction

There are two things that you must do to pass the examinations for the diploma of the FFARCS: you must reach a certain level of knowledge; and you must know how to present it to the examiners. This is the second of two books that are more concerned with the latter requirement; they will also help you to assess your level of knowledge, but they should not be treated as sources of knowledge.

In the first book of 600 MCQs we set questions on physiology, pharmacology and clinical measurement. This book covers a full range of clinical topics on which you may be questioned in both the written and oral sections of Parts I and III of the examination: these include medicine, surgery, applied pharmacology, anatomy, and both general and specialised questions on anaesthesia and intensive care.

The standard textbooks are the best source books of basic knowledge for the FFARCS. The more specialised texts, reviews in the journals, and discussion with others should be used to build upon this knowledge — to update it and to find faults in it. You cannot expect to pass an exam unless you work for it: the more clinically oriented is the exam, then the more importance you must place on gaining wide experience in clinical anaesthesia. You must avoid the danger of working too much 'at the books'.

Many people think that the key to these exams is to go on a course, and there is no doubt that courses can be extremely useful. They should, however, be thought of as a means of aiming one's studies in the right directions; it is disappointing to find that many people will attend a course 2–3 months before the hurdle of a major examination apparently without having done any work. This is foolhardy. To get the most out of a course, one should have covered some of the groundwork beforehand. Once you have acquired what you hope to be sufficient knowledge (and in the absence of a published syllabus this must sometimes be a matter of guesswork in some areas), then is the time that these books should be of help to you.

HOW TO ANSWER MULTIPLE CHOICE QUESTIONS

The format of the MCQs in the FFA examination is a stem and five branches. The stem may be short ('Mitral stenosis causes:'), or may be a few lines, for example when presenting a clinical problem. Each of the five branches that follow may be true or false. You score one mark for each correct answer, minus one for each incorrect answer, and, extremely important to the exam technique, you score nothing if you choose not to answer a particular branch. Your actual answers are marked by computer, and so you must eventually but them onto special cards that are supplied separately. These cards have the question numbers printed on them and you indicate your answer by filling in a 'true' or a 'false' box in pencil.

The most important tactic is not to guess: if you don't know — leave that branch blank. You should also think very carefully if you think a branch (or a stem) is ambiguous.

You must read each stem very carefully: watch out for qualifying words such as 'commonly', 'rarely', 'always', and the like because they can turn what would otherwise be a 'false' into a 'true' and vice versa. Re-read the stem with each statement: it is all too easy to forget the emphasis and exact wording of the stem as you work down the five branches. Watch out for negatives: in the heat of the moment you may fail to see 'not' in a branch. 'May' is an awkward word; one can argue that anything 'may' cause anything else. Try to give the answer relevant to clinical practice: for instance, it is 'true' that atropine may cause bradycardia, but not that propranolol may relieve bronchospasm.

It is impossible to write an MCQ paper without some of the questions being ambiguous or some of the answers being arguable. This is more likely in the applied clinical subjects than in the basic sciences because questions can be less clearly matters of fact, and may be matters of opinion. We apologise for this, but some of the questions in the actual exam paper will be ambiguous, or will seem so to you in the examination hall, and you must learn how to deal with them.

It is easier when compiling MCQ questions to think of true branches than of false branches, which must appear to some candidates to be true or else the question will not discriminate between the good candidate and the poor one. False branches are sometimes complete red herrings. These can be very difficult to answer and you may not be able to find the correct answer in the literature because the connection does not exist.

Clinical questions in MCQ examinations commonly give a short clinical scenario in which the stem is a truncated history with perhaps the results of a few investigations. The branches may ask, for instance, for 'possible' or 'probable' diagnoses. The papers in this book include some questions of this type, but there is no substitute for clinical experience, and that is the best way of improving your performance on applied clinical questions.

A STRATEGY FOR A MULTIPLE CHOICE PAPER

You should have a general strategy for answering an MCQ paper.

For those who haven't, we suggest one here. We are not saying it is the only one, but we think it allows efficient use of the time spent answering the paper.

First, read through the questions from the first to the last, answering quickly those of which you are certain of the answers. Mark the options T or F on the question paper; it is not a good idea to mark the computer card as you go because it is then not as easy to check your answers.

You will probably find that you can tell from the stem whether or not you will be able to answer a question. If you cannot answer a question immediately on this first read-through, put a question mark by it if you will need to think about it (and by any answers of which you are a little uncertain), and put a cross against those that you think you will probably not be able to answer at all. It is very important not to dwell on doubtful questions at all first time through or you may find yourself short of time before you have answered all the questions that you DO know.

On the second read-through, tackle those that you marked with a question mark; don't be afraid to scribble notes on scrap paper to help you with confusing questions. After this second read-through it is worth going back and checking the answers — but don't dwell on those that you answered on the first read-through or you will find yourself doubting even your most cast-iron certainties. At this stage, transfer the answers that you have made so far to the computer cards AND MAKE SURE THAT YOU MARK THE CARDS CORRECTLY; it is easy to get out of phase between the question numbers and answer numbers. You should now regard these answers as immutable: don't look at the questions again and get on with answering those that you marked with a cross. Answers to these questions you can mark on the computer cards right away because you will have had plenty to time to think around the subject.

When you have answered all you can, check that you have written your name everywhere that you should have done, and it may be better to leave the examination hall. With essay questions, you should always be able to add more to your answers, and you should stay for every precious minute; staying and staring at MCQ answers induces neurosis.

THE MCQ PAPERS IN THIS BOOK

The 600 questions are arranged in 10 'papers' of 60 questions with each 'paper' containing questions on a mix of subjects. In the actual examination, approximately 2 minutes are allowed for each question, but this time includes the time needed to transfer your answers to the cards. We suggest that the best way to test yourself is to try a whole 'paper' under examination conditions, unseen, in one and a half to one and three-quarter hours. If you take longer than this you may run out of time in the exam when transferring your answers. The index at the back of the book allows access to the questions under broad subject headings so that you could, if you wanted, answer a number of questions from different papers on, say, respiratory medicine. You will, however, gain nothing if you look at the answers without trying the questions; and there is little to gain from trying a question if you have not done the work on the subject. There are more questions on some topics than on others. Some of the questions in the later papers on these important topics are similar to the questions in earlier papers and will allow you to assess whether your understanding of the topic has improved.

HOW TO SCORE YOURSELF

For each branch, score +1 if you marked correctly True or False, or −1 if you marked incorrectly True or False. Score nil for any branch for which you gave no answer. The maximum for each question is thus +5, and the minimum is −5.

Your overall score on a 'paper' will give some idea of your general level of knowledge, bearing in mind that you may not be tested on all the subjects included here in the MCQ paper (though they are fair game in essays or vivas) and that Part III now includes physics with clinical measurement. We cannot say what score corresponds to a 'pass' in the MCQ in the actual exam, but, from our experience of setting mock papers to candidates in the past, you should be looking for 40% to 50%, and 60% to 70% is a good score.

As well as your overall score it is worth calculating your 'efficiency ratio', which is the number of correct answers expressed as a percentage of the total number of attempted answers. Thus you can get an overall score of 50% by answering 150 branches correctly (an efficiency of 100%) or by answering 190 but getting 20 of them wrong: 170 × (+1) minus 20 × (−1). A low total score with a high efficiency implies that you are certain of what you know but that your overall knowledge is not enough; a low efficiency ratio means that your knowledge is faulty, or that you are guessing.

Often, candidates going up for the exam ask how many branches they should aim to answer. The only sensible answer to this is that you should answer all that you can. There is no 'safe' number. Certainly, if you are able only to answer 40%, then that is unlikely to be enough to pass, but merely ploughing on and guessing to bring your total answered up above 50% is unlikely to increase your score because half of your additional answers, if they are pure guesses, will be incorrect. Similarly, if you have answered 60%, don't assume that there is no need to answer any more — you may have answered incorrectly more than you think.

Your overall score will indicate your knowledge; your efficiency ratio will point out gross faults in technique of answering; you should also look very carefully at those individual questions at which you scored badly. Using the same reasoning as for the complete paper, you will need to score 3 out of 5 to 'pass' a single question. Think carefully why you did poorly on a particular question. The usual reason is simply lack of knowledge and occasionally you will find a complete gap such that you are unable to answer any of the branches of a question. A very high negative score (−4 or −5) usually implies a lack of understanding of the question rather than lack of knowledge, or a misunderstanding of the wording. These high negative scores have a great effect on your overall score and perhaps one of the major lessons of this book is to help you to avoid them. As we have stressed before, it is essential to read each question very carefully: don't rush at the questions.

THE ANSWERS AND COMMENTS

In the answer section for each paper we give explanations of the correct answers and also make comments, if appropriate, on the form and wording of the question. It is very easy to become side-tracked and obsessed when you get a particular branch wrong which you feel you marked correctly: you may find a source which shows you are indeed correct. However, nobody fails the MCQ paper because of one branch that, according to the 'correct' answer, they answered incorrectly — concentrate instead on those questions on which you did badly overall. If you scored −3 on a question about thyroid disease it would be more valuable to go and read a good account of the thyroid, and to seek help from others, than to feel aggrieved that you think we are wrong on one particular point and waste time laboriously checking each particular branch.

We cannot give full explanations for all the branches in all the questions: that would mean writing a series of large textbooks. Some questions demand more explanation than others and some questions have very short comments. In general, false branches get more explanation than do true ones. The length of the explanation given has no bearing necessarily on the importance of the topic. For some of the more important topics we advise you to consult the textbooks if you do badly. There are no references quoted, but it should be possible to answer all the questions in the book from reading the standard texts.

THE LAST WORD

The examiners try to set questions on sensible, mainstream, subjects that are clear and unambiguous. They are not trying to be devious and trick you into giving incorrect answers. It is often said that MCQs are unfair because they penalise the candidate who has read widely and who can always find a reason why 'true' is actually 'sometimes true' or 'maybe true'. MCQs have to have black-or-white answers: when testing basic knowledge or general principles, what the examiner wants to know is whether the candidate can see the wood for the trees.

Contents

Paper I Questions

I.1 Suitable constituents of a cardioplegic solution for coronary vein bypass grafting include:

A potassium
B bicarbonate
C glucagon
D dextrose
E procaine.

I.2 A 50-year-old woman presents for emergency surgery with acute dyspnoea caused by a huge goitre. She is clinically euthyroid and seems otherwise fit. Your management would include:

A a tracheostomy under local anaesthetic before surgery
B Lugol's iodine prior to induction
C blind nasal intubation after adequate preoxygenation, intravenous induction and suxamethonium
D the use of an armoured endotracheal tube
E thoracic inlet views.

I.3 Contra-indications to outpatient general anaesthesia in the dental chair include:

A upper respiratory tract infection
B trismus
C sickle-cell disease
D epilepsy
E angina.

I.4 A 4-year-old boy is brought back to the operating theatre at 18.00 h because he is continuing to bleed following a tonsillectomy that morning. He is restless and obviously in some discomfort. His pulse is 145, his BP 85/60:

A he should have premedication to calm him before induction
B he should be induced with an inhalational agent
C you would make attempts to empty the stomach once he is anaesthetized
D you would ask the surgeon to secure haemostasis under local anaesthesia because of the risk of a general anaesthetic
E you would insert an intravenous cannula prior to induction.

I.5 Techniques of topical anaesthesia suitable for nasal surgery include:

A Moffet's method
B the use of cocaine paste
C Krause's method
D packing with 20% cocaine in adrenaline
E Bodman's method.

I.6 A suitable anaesthetic technique for squint correction in a 5-year-old child would include:

A the avoidance of of intramuscular atropine
B halothane
C intermittent positive pressure ventilation
D endotracheal intubation
E opiate premedication.

I.7 Failure to maintain antihypertensive therapy up to the day of operation:

A leads to hypokalaemia during operation
B causes severe hypertension post-operatively
C impairs renal function during surgery
D is associated with exaggerated blood pressure responses to noxious stimuli
E is associated with episodes of myocardial ischaemia during surgery.

I.8 Delayed recovery of consciousness following general anaesthesia may be caused by:

A intra-operative hypoxia
B carbon dioxide narcosis
C heavy preoperative medication with narcotic analgesics
D residual curarization
E hyperventilation.

I.9 Common immediate problems of laryngoscopy and intubation include:

A hypotension
B dysrhythmias in more than 50% of patients
C dislocation of the arytenoid cartilages
D bronchospasm
E surgical emphysema due to pharyngeal trauma.

I.10 Patients likely to develop adult respiratory distress syndrome include those suffering from:

A severe abdominal sepsis
B renal failure
C haemorrhagic shock
D prolonged high-concentration oxygen therapy
E burns to the limbs and trunk.

I.11 Intermittent mandatory ventilation:

A is useful in neonatal resuscitation
B is useful in weaning patients from artificial ventilation
C is achieved by inducing rebreathing
D is a means whereby a patient can breathe spontaneously with occasional assisted breaths
E is a method of triggering spontaneous breaths.

I.12 Spread of local anaesthetic solution within the epidural space is influenced by:

A posture
B degree of obesity
C pregnancy
D speed of injection
E age.

I.13 The following endotracheal tubes would be suitable for use in neurosurgical anaesthesia:

A Oxford
B Magill red rubber
C Bart's model flexometallic
D Bryce-Smith
E Portex.

I.14 The following are contra-indicated in closed head injury:

A 25 g mannitol intravenously
B homatropine eyedrops
C morphine
D general anaesthesia with spontaneous respiration
E phenobarbitone.

I.15 To minimize the risk of acid regurgitation and Mendelson's syndrome in a patient presenting for Caesarian section, one should:

A administer an antacid pre-operatively
B induce anaesthesia in the left lateral position
C apply cricoid pressure prior to and during endotracheal intubation
D induce vomiting beforehand with apomorphine
E apply topical anaesthesia to the larynx.

I.16 Indications for the use of lumbar epidural anaesthesia during labour include:

A placenta praevia
B eclampsia
C prematurity
D cardiac valvular disease
E maternal exhaustion.

I.17 The following are true of cystic fibrosis:

A it is inherited as an autosomal recessive
B it is one of the rarest of the inherited conditions
C it is a condition specifically of the mucous glands of the respiratory tract
D diagnosis can be confirmed by finding a raised sodium concentration in sweat
E daily prophylactic antibiotics are a sensible precaution against chest infection.

I.18 Chronic conditions likely to benefit from sympathetic blockade include:

A causalgia
B trigeminal neuralgia
C Raynaud's disease
D phantom limb pain
E pain associated with pancreatic carcinoma.

I.19 Soda lime:

A contains 70% calcium hydroxide and 30% sodium hydroxide
B may warm up to 60°C during active carbon dioxide absorption
C produces humidification of inspired gases
D is contra-indicated if enflurane is being used
E 100 g provides approximately 1 hour of absorbing capacity.

I.20 The action of d-tubocurarine is enhanced by:

A liver failure
B hypokalaemia
C gentamicin administration
D metabolic acidosis
E hypercapnoea.

I.21 Appropriate therapy for severe hypertension occurring following intravenous ephedrine administration in a patient on chronic tranylcypromine therapy includes:

A propanolol
B phentolamine
C diazoxide
D guanethidine
E reserpine.

I.22 Appropriate treatment of a patient thought to have suffered an anaphylactic response to thiopentone would include:

A intravenous hydrocortisone
B subcutaneous adrenaline
C volume expansion with dextran
D intravenous cimetidine
E intravenous chlorpheniramine.

I.23 The Carlens double lumen endobronchial tube:

A is only suitable for intubation of the left main bronchus
B has a carinal hook
C was not originally designed for endobronchial anaesthesia
D has its two lumens lying one in front of the other for extra rigidity
E has a double endobronchial cuff.

I.24 A patient presents for left thoracotomy and resection of a large lung cyst. During anaesthesia:

A nitrous oxide is contra-indicated
B intermittent positive pressure ventilation should be avoided until the cyst has been isolated from the bronchial tree
C halothane is a suitable anaesthetic
D endobronchial intubation is contra-indicated
E topical endobronchial anaesthesia should not be used.

I.25 The following are true of the anatomy of the large airways:

A the tracheal bifurcation is at the level of the 4th to 6th thoracic vertebrae in the adult
B the different angles of branching of the main bronchi are exaggerated in children
C the right main bronchus is about 2.5 cm long in the adult
D each lung normally has 10 bronchopulmonary segments
E the right main bronchus is related to the azygos vein.

I.26 Concerning the nerve supply to the arm:

A the radial nerve supplies flexors of the wrist
B the radial nerve supplies skin on the opposing surfaces of the thumb and index finger
C the median nerve passes deep to the bicipital aponeurosis
D the radial nerve supplies skin over the back of the elbow
E the only motor fibres in the ulnar nerve are to small muscles in the hand.

I.27 The diaphragm:

A takes its origin from the last six costal cartilages
B is inserted into the first three lumbar vertebrae via the crura
C from anterior to posterior is traversed by the oesophagus, inferior vena cava and aorta
D moves up to 10 cm or more in deep inspiration
E comes up to the level of the 5th rib in the mid-axillary line.

I.28 In the intercostal spaces:

A the external intercostal muscle runs down and forwards
B the nerves lie superficial to posterior intercostal arteries beneath the corresponding rib
C the posterior intercostal arteries are branches of the internal mammary artery
D about 3 ml of a suitable local anaesthetic solution will effect blockade of each nerve
E the inner surface anteriorly is formed by the parietal pleura.

I.29 The maxillary division of the trigeminal nerve subserves sensation from:

A the skin over the temple
B the bridge of the nose
C the maxillary sinus
D the upper teeth
E the upper lip.

I.30 The following are true of the nerve supply to the leg:

A the upper inner aspect of the thigh is supplied by the ilio-inguinal and genito-femoral nerves
B the obturator nerve supplies a constant area over the medial aspect of the thigh
C the anterior division of the femoral nerve is a purely sensory nerve
D the posterior division of the femoral nerve supplies the quadriceps muscle and ends as the saphenous nerve
E sensation from the knee joint is subserved by the sciatic, femoral and obturator nerves.

I.31 Concerning the recurrent laryngeal nerve:

A in organic palsy, the abductors are paralysed first
B unilateral palsies cause complete aphonia
C the left has a longer intrathoracic course than the right
D temporary paralysis may occur during stellate ganglion block
E bilateral paralysis is an absolute indication for tracheostomy.

I.32 Causes of a primary metabolic acidosis include:

A vomiting
B hydronephrosis
C hypokalaemia
D diabetes mellitus
E intestinal fistulae.

I.33 Hyponatraemia with total body depletion of sodium occurs in:

A refractory heart failure with dependent pitting oedema
B diabetic ketoacidosis
C water intoxication
D Addisonian crisis
E renal failure.

I.34 Causes of a hyperdynamic circulation include:

A anaemia
B myxoedema
C pregnancy
D Paget's disease
E pulmonary embolism.

I.35 A 57-year-old man is admitted to hospital following a myocardial infarction. The ECG shows ST elevation in leads II, III and aVF, and ST depression in lead I. His blood pressure is 120/90 mm Hg. Catheterization reveals PAP 30/60 mm Hg, PCWP 25 mm Hg, RAP 8 cm H_2O, CVP +10 cm H_2O. The following are consistent with this clinical situation:

A tricuspid regurgitation
B left ventricular failure
C left ventricular failure with fluid overload
D simple fluid overload
E right ventricular failure plus left ventricular failure.

I.36 A third heart sound:

A is a normal occurrence in young people
B is present in left ventricular failure
C is associated with mitral stenosis
D occurs in constrictive pericarditis
E occurs during systole.

I.37 Acute cardiac tamponade is associated with:

A massive ascites
B increased 'a' waves on the jugular venous pressure wave
C bradycardia
D cyanosis and peripheral shutdown
E pulsus paradoxus.

I.38 The following conditions make the accidental intravenous injection of a small volume of air a particular hazard:

A ventricular septal defect
B pulmonary stenosis
C tricuspid regurgitation
D patent ductus arteriosus
E atrial septal defect.

I.39 In diabetes mellitus:

A insulin requirements decrease in pregnancy
B there is an increased incidence of renal papillary necrosis
C postural hypotension occurs
D serial glucose tolerance tests are used in assessing treatment
E retinopathy is an early complication.

I.40 In a patient with acute intermittent porphyria in whom a crisis is precipitated, associated symptoms include:

A coma
B paralysis
C skin lesions
D tinnitus
E mania.

I.41 The following drugs cause convulsions:

A benzyl penicillin
B methohexitone
C primidone
D insulin
E overtransfusion with 5% dextrose.

I.42 Likely complications of ulcerative colitis include:

A anaemia
B acute toxic colonic dilation
C perforation
D hypocalcaemia
E hypoproteinaemia.

I.43 Chronic constipation is a complication of:

A hyperthyroidism
B hyperkalaemia
C porphyria
D hypercalcaemia
E autonomic neuropathy.

I.44 Portal hypertension occurs with:
- **A** hepatic venous thrombosis
- **B** constrictive pericarditis
- **C** tricuspid incompetence
- **D** biliary cirrhosis
- **E** polycythaemia.

I.45 The development of disseminated intravascular coagulation is associated with:
- **A** cardiac surgery
- **B** prostatic carcinoma
- **C** head injury
- **D** parturition
- **E** haemophilia.

I.46 Reticulocytosis is seen in:
- **A** acute leukaemia
- **B** treated vitamin B_{12} deficiency
- **C** haemolytic anaemia
- **D** sickle-cell disease
- **E** thalassaemia.

I.47 Typical anticholinergic effects include:
- **A** dry mouth
- **B** increased gastro-intestinal motility
- **C** bradycardia
- **D** increased sweating
- **E** bronchodilation.

I.48 Metoclopramide:
- **A** is useful for opiate-induced nausea
- **B** is not so effective if given after atropine
- **C** has only a peripheral action
- **D** does not cause extrapyramidal side-effects
- **E** can be given orally or intramuscularly.

I.49 The following are features of chronic renal failure:
- **A** bleeding tendency
- **B** macrocytic anaemia
- **C** hypertension
- **D** splenomegaly
- **E** tetany.

I.50 On a chest radiograph:

A the right diaphragm is usually at a higher level than the left
B Kerley's B lines represent the superior pulmonary veins
C the lesser fissure is usually at the level of the 6th rib in the axilla
D a pneumothorax is best demonstrated on an inspiratory film
E the carina is at the level of T4.

I.51 Prolonged cigarette smoking is associated with the development of:

A oesophageal carcinoma
B myocardial ischaemia
C Buerger's disease
D peptic ulceration
E hyperglycaemia.

I.52 Clinical signs commonly observed in a chronic bronchitic suffering from acute respiratory failure include

A small volume pulse
B cold extremities
C elevated jugular venous pressure
D tremor
E papilloedema.

I.53 Conditions associated with pathological cyanosis include:

A polycythaemia
B asthma
C pulmonary consolidation
D mitral valve disease
E methaemoglobinaemia.

I.54 Likely causes of surgical emphysema in a patient with vomiting, abdominal pain and dyspnoea include:

A pulmonary infarction
B ruptured diaphragm
C spontaneous pneumothorax
D ruptured oesophagus
E ruptured trachea.

I.55 Tumours of the salivary glands:

A are commonest in the parotid glands
B are most commonly a pleomorphic adenoma
C are usually malignant but slow-growing
D when malignant tend to be radio-resistant
E should be biopsied before surgery.

I.56 Primary malignant tumours which commonly metastasize to lung include:

A testicular seminoma
B thyroid carcinoma
C ovarian carcinoma
D hypernephroma
E breast carcinoma.

I.57 Cholangiocarcinoma:

A is commoner in young women taking the contraceptive pill
B presents with symptoms of obstructive jaundice
C is associated with gallstones
D is associated with alcoholism
E may be cured by a Whipple's operation.

I.58 The following are true of carcinoma of the stomach:

A it is commoner in men and especially those between 40 and 60 years of age
B it is associated with achlorhydria
C a longer history is associated with a better prognosis
D a curative operation must remove the whole stomach
E palliative radiotherapy is useful.

I.59 Complications of a Colles fracture include:

A drop wrist
B median nerve damage
C late rupture of tendons at the wrist
D avascular necrosis of the radial fragment
E Dupuytren's contracture.

I.60 Hypernephroma:

A is an adenocarcinoma
B is particularly likely to spread via the venous system
C presents most commonly as painless haematuria
D is a cause of pyrexia of unknown origin
E is a contra-indication to retrograde pyelography.

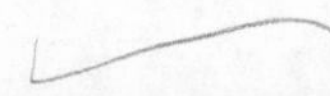

Paper I Answers

I.1 **TTFTT**

C Glucagon is an inotrope and therefore undesirable.
E Procaine acts as a membrane stabilizer.

I.2 **FFFTT**

A If the goitre is 'huge', the trachea will be behind it.
B Lugol's iodine takes days to have effect.
C An awake intubation is required, and an oral tube is satisfactory. It doesn't have to be armoured (**D**), but some anaesthetists like them.

I.3 **TTTTT**

Patients for outpatient general anaesthesia in the dental chair should be completely fit and healthy.

I.4 **FTTFT**

A,B These are arguable but, whatever is done, one must remember that the patient may be severely hypovolaemic. He should be resuscitated, transfused if necessary, prior to induction (**E**).
C There is likely to be a stomach full of blood.
D Perhaps in an adult, certainly not in a 4-year-old.

I.5 **TTFFT**

A,C,E If you quote the eponymous names then you must expect to be asked the details of the techniques.

C This method is used to anaesthetize the internal laryngeal nerve in the pyriform fossae.

D The cocaine concentration is too high — 10% maximum.

I.6 **FTTTT**

A There is no need to avoid atropine in this situation, though one might choose to give it intravenously at induction: one should do something to obtund the oculocardiac reflex.

I.7 **FTFTT**

A,C No reason why it should.

I.8 **TTTFT**

D This does not affect level of consciousness.

I.9 **FFFFF**

A–E Be careful — while all of these are documented, the question asked for COMMON, IMMEDIATE complications.

B Dysrhythmias occur, but 50% incidence is too high.

I.10 **TFTTT**

B Renal failure is not associated with ARDS unless both have been caused by, for example, severe trauma.

I.11 FTFTF

C There should be no rebreathing in an IMV circuit.
E No — it is a method whereby spontaneous and ventilated breaths are synchronized, but no triggering is involved.

I.12 TFTTT

B Although it may affect the dose, it doesn't affect the spread.

I.13 TFTFT

B Kinks.
C This tube has no bevel.
D Red herring — this is a double lumen tube.
E Often used, but will still kink, particularly when warm.

I.14 FTTTF

A Will lower ICP by promoting an osmotic diuresis.
B,C Any drug that affects pupillary diameter masks neurological evaluation.
D May cause hypercarbia, cerebral vasodilation and a rise in ICP.
E Often used to reduce cerebral metabolic rate and "protect" the brain.

I.15 TFTFF

B One can, but it isn't usually done and (**C**) is a better precaution.
D Cruel and little used.
E Contra-indicated because it makes the larynx incompetent.

I.16 FTTTT

A Although placenta praevia may not be a contra-indication in some cases, the question asks specifically for INDICATIONS. In addition, placenta praevia may be associated with considerable blood loss and hypotension.
D It was once held that cardiac disease (the commonest problem in this age group being rheumatic mitral disease) was a contra-indication.

I.17 TFFTT

B It is one of the commonest of the inherited conditions in Great Britain (about one in 2–3000 live births).

C It affects mucus- and non-mucus-secreting glands, affecting mainly pancreas and lungs.

E *Staph. aureus* infections are particularly feared, and many authorities suggest daily flucloxacillin.

I.18 TFTTT

B There is no sympathetic involvement in this condition.

I.19 FTTFT

A 90% calcium hydroxide, 5% sodium hydroxide.

D Not incompatible with enflurane.

I.20 FTTTT

A Not sufficient metabolism to produce a clinical effect.

I.21 TTTFF

The question says 'severe' and implies acute hypertension following ephedrine in a patient on MAOIs.

C Probably reasonable, as it acts directly.

D,E Indirect and slow-acting — inappropriate.

I.22 TTFFT

C Volume expansion is important: remember that dextran itself can be a cause of anaphylaxis.

D H_2 receptor blockade is unnecessary.

I.23 TTTFF

A The comparable right-sided tube is a White.

C Was originally used for bronchopulmonary spirometry.

D The lumens are side by side, as in a Robertshaw.

E This idea is only present on the Brompton 'triple cuff' endobronchial tube.

I.24 TTTFF

D Endobronchial intubation may be essential.

E There is no reason why not.

I.25 TFTFT

A The level varies with posture and lung volume.

B The angles are more equal in children.

D The left lung normally has nine segments.

I.26 FFTTF

A Radial palsy = wrist drop because of unopposed flexion.

B Skin on the back of the hand, not the opposing surfaces.

E Long flexors as well.

I.27 **TTFTT**

B The normal anatomy has insertion on the right into L1–3 and on the left into L1–2.

C From anterior to posterior: IVC — oesophagus — aorta.

E The 5th rib laterally is at the same level as the 8th vertebra posteriorly.

I.28 **TTFTT**

C The anterior intercostals (which anastomose with the posterior intercostals) arise from the internal mammary.

E The innermost intercostal muscle is the inner surface posteriorly, but ends at the anterior axillary line.

I.29 **TFTTT**

B The frontal branch of the ophthalmic division.

I.30 **TFFTT**

B The relative contributions of the medial cutaneous (femoral), obturator, and saphenous (femoral) nerves is variable.

C Motor as well, including sartorius.

I.31 **TFTTF**

B Only hoarseness.

E Very few things are 'absolute', although tracheostomy may indeed be required.

I.32 FTFTT

A Vomiting causes a metabolic alkalosis.
C Hypokalaemia induces an intracellular acidosis and produces a metabolic alkalosis.

I.33 FFFTT

A There is sodium retention in heart failure.
B The patient is likely to be dehydrated and therefore hypernatraemic.
C Total body sodium is diluted when there is water overload.
E Not all renal failure is salt-losing.

I.34 TFTTF

B Low output state and reduced metabolic rate.
D Patients develop arteriovenous fistulae in abnormal bone.
E Low output due to obstructed pulmonary blood flow.

I.35 FTFFF

Look at the stem and think: probably an inferior infarct; not shocked; low PA diastolic pressure and a high wedge pressure. The correct answers follow from this consideration. Incidentally, the clinical history and ECG findings are perhaps an indication for catheterization, but are irrelevant to the consideration of the results.

I.36 TTFTF

C,E A third heart sound occurs during diastole and is associated with either tricuspid or mitral regurgitation.

I.37 FTFTT

A Although the two may occur together, this is not a common association.
C Tachycardia, due to circulatory failure.
D Because of the circulatory failure.

I.38 TFFTT

The danger is an arterial embolus of air, so any right-to-left connection is a hazard even though, with normal haemodynamics, flow would be from left to right through the defects.

I.39 FTTFF

A In pregnancy, insulin requirements increase, the renal threshold for glucose decreases.

D Useful in diagnosis but not in the assessment of treatment.

E Not an early complication. It occurs in juvenile-onset diabetics when they reach middle age.

I.40 TTFFT

C Skin lesions are not a feature of an acute crisis.

D Tinnitus sounds plausible but is not a typical feature.

I.41 TTFTT

A Penicillin can cause convulsions either in extreme overdose or if given intrathecally.

C An anticonvulsant with a structure similar to phenobarbitone.

D Hypoglycaemic convulsions (the now outdated 'insulin shock therapy').

I.42 TTTFT

D Calcium is not absorbed or secreted in the large bowel.

I.43 FFTTT

A Hyperthyroidism causes diarrhoea.

B Hypokalaemia causes constipation.

I.44 TTFTT

C Tricuspid stenosis will cause an extrahepatic, post-sinusoidal portal hypertension.

E Polycythaemia precipitates portal venous thrombosis.

I.45 TFTTF

B Some malignancies, e.g. lung, but not prostate — prostatic carcinoma is associated with abnormal fibrinolysis.

I.46 FTTTF

Reticulocytosis indicates increased production of red cells. The count is reduced in acute leukaemia (**A**).

E Thalassaemia is not a single entity and the blood findings vary according to the variety, but there is no reticulocytosis.

I.47 TFFFT

B Reduced motility.

C Tachycardia.

D Dry skin, sweating inhibited.

I.48 TTFFT

B Atropine counters the peripheral action of metoclopramide.

C Also has a central action.

D Particularly likely in patients with renal failure, for unknown reasons.

I.49 TFTFF

A Coagulation factors and platelet function are abnormal.

B Normochromic, normocytic anaemia is likely.

E Patients are hypocalcaemic for a number of reasons, but tetany is rare.

I.50 TFTFT

B 'B' lines are basal, horizontal and indicate increased lung water. They occur when there is raised left atrial pressure.

D Expiratory films are better for showing pneumothorax.

I.51 TTTFF

D Although the mortality from peptic ulcer is increased, the incidence is not.

E Hypoglycaemia sometimes occurs as an idiosyncratic response.

I.52 FFFTT

The question implies acute carbon dioxide retention.

A,B CO_2 retention produces a good volume pulse and vasodilation.

C These patients are often oedematous because of sodium and bicarbonate retention without being in right heart failure: the question does not imply heart failure.

I.53 TTTTT

I.54 FFTTF

A,B Not associated with surgical emphysema.

E Very unlikely except as a result of direct trauma.

I.55 TTFTF

B The mixed parotid tumour, for example.

C They are usually slow-growing, but benign.

E Salivary tumours tend to seed if biopsied or handled roughly at operation. Whether to biopsy depends on the site and likelihood of malignancy, but should be done with caution.

I.56 **TTFTT**

Note inclusion of the word 'commonly'.

C Transperitoneal spread.

I.57 **FTTFF**

A Hepatomas have been described (rarely) in women on the pill.

E Whipple's operation is for carcinoma of the head of pancreas. Curative operation for cholangiocarcinoma is extremely unlikely.

I.58 **TTTFF**

C This sounds paradoxical, but is because the prognosis depends on the histology.

D The amount of stomach to be resected for cure (when possible) depends on the site of the tumour (which determines its lymphatic drainage).

E Adenocarcinomas are resistant to radiotherapy.

I.59 **FTTFF**

A The radial nerve carries no motor supply at this level and is unlikely to be damaged anyway.

D Avascular necrosis is recognized following fractures of the scaphoid, not of the radius.

E Totally unconnected: Volkmann's ischaemic contracture is a complication.

I.60 **TTTTF**

B Tumour tends to grow into the renal veins.

E Retrograde pyelography is extremely useful.

Paper II Questions

II.1 Appropriate anaesthetic techniques for cardiac catheterization in children include:

A rectal thiopentone
B intramuscular diazepam
C ketamine
D oxygen and halothane
E trichloroethylene and air.

II.2 Contra-indications to general anaesthesia in the dental chair include:

A steroid therapy
B diabetes mellitus
C dental abscess
D mental retardation
E anaphylaxis to local anaesthetic agents.

II.3 A 69-year-old man is to undergo laryngectomy for a glottic tumour that is causing obstructed breathing. He is taking beta-blockers for hypertension. He smokes 30 cigarettes a day. The following are true:

A a pre-operative chest X-ray is not needed if he has no symptoms referable to the lower respiratory tract
B intra-arterial monitoring of blood pressure is justifiable
C a monitor of central venous pressure is mandatory
D a rapid sequence intravenous induction, aided by an introducer down the endotracheal tube, would be a sensible approach
E the patient should be ventilated post-operatively.

II.4 The following vaporisers are not temperature-compensated:

A Boyle's bottle
B Oxford miniature vaporiser (OMV)
C copper kettle
D E.M.O.
E Goldman.

II.5 Appropriate drugs for use during general anaesthesia for cataract extraction in an 80-year-old man include:

A suxamethonium
B pancuronium
C promethazine
D halothane
E atropine.

II.6 Concerning the stages of anaesthesia:

A these were first described by Guedel with reference to ether anaesthesia
B stage 2 is the stage of excitement
C intercostal paralysis is complete in plane 3 of stage 3
D regular automatic respiration commences in plane 1 of stage 3
E there is no respiratory response to skin incision in stage 3.

II.7 If oral intubation is found to be extremely difficult in an emergency case, in which suxamethonium has already been administered, a correct course of action would be to:

A continue to attempt oral intubation until successful
B hand-ventilate with a face mask while maintaining cricoid pressure
C perform emergency tracheostomy
D attempt blind nasal intubation
E restore normal spontaneous ventilation and summon assistance.

II.8 Carbon dioxide production is:

A reduced by halothane
B increased by parenteral nutrition
C increased during convulsions
D increased by acetazolamide
E independent of the state of consciousness.

II.9 In the development of gram-negative septic shock:

A circulating endotoxin causes the release of chemical mediators which increase vascular permeability
B lack of ATP results in failure of the sodium pump
C septicaemia may result from instrumentation of the biliary tree
D the fibrinolytic system is not involved
E steroids maintain the stability of lysosomal membranes.

II.10 Intermittent positive pressure ventilation is likely to be needed postoperatively if the patient:

A has an arterial pCO_2 of 80 mm Hg (10.7 kPa)
B has an arterial pO_2 of 60 mm Hg (8.0 kPa)
C has pain on coughing
D has a vital capacity of only 2 litres
E cannot hold his breath for more than 10 seconds.

II.11 Stellate ganglion block produces:

- **A** hoarseness
- **B** ipsilateral mydriasis
- **C** enophthalmos
- **D** anaesthesia of the supraglottic larynx
- **E** increased cerebral blood flow.

II.12 In an unconscious patient, thought to be suffering from a ruptured intracranial aneurysm, anaesthesia for carotid angiography:

- **A** should include hyperventilation
- **B** is best achieved with a spontaneously breathing patient
- **C** should commence with a 'crash' induction
- **D** should include elective induced hypotension
- **E** should be preceded by intravenous atropine.

II.13 In a patient with traumatic quadriplegia of one week's duration, likely problems include:

- **A** hypotension resulting from IPPV
- **B** adductor spasm of the legs
- **C** increased resistance to suxamethonium
- **D** hyperthermia
- **E** bladder distension.

II.14 Relaxation of the pregnant uterus is rapidly achieved with:

- **A** spinal anaesthesia
- **B** nitrous oxide
- **C** trichloroethylene
- **D** halothane
- **E** amyl nitrite.

II.15 Contra-indications to the use of lumbar epidural anaesthesia during labour include:

- **A** previous Caesarian section
- **B** fetal distress
- **C** maternal haemorrhagic tendency
- **D** breech delivery
- **E** eclampsia.

II.16 Concerning the Ayre's T-piece circuit:

- **A** the internal diameter of the reservoir tube should be 1 cm
- **B** the fresh gas flow for a child of 6 months breathing spontaneously should be 5 l/min
- **C** there is a reservoir tube of sufficient capacity to prevent rebreathing
- **D** the tidal volume of a 10 kg child is 60–70 ml
- **E** during spontaneous ventilation, fresh gas flow should be at least twice the patient's minute volume.

II.17 Likely complications of the use of epidural opioid for post-operative analgesia include:

A itching
B hypotension
C hypoventilation
D sedation
E urinary retention.

II.18 Concerning anaesthetic potency:

A the MAC for halothane in humans without nitrous oxide is 0.765%
B although the saturated vapour pressure of methoxyflurane is low, the MAC implies that it is a potent anaesthetic agent
C in the methane series of hydrocarbon molecules, potency increases as chlorine replaces fluorine
D non-rebreathing anaesthetic systems induce anaesthesia more slowly than closed systems
E rate of induction with a soluble agent such as ether is increased by hyperventilation

II.19 Thiopentone:

A forms a precipitate if mixed with suxamethonium
B may induce acute demyelination and paralysis in patients with porphyria
C induces its own hepatic metabolism
D is an analgesic
E is a sulphur analogue of pentobarbitone.

II.20 The following cause pupillary dilatation:

A intravenous neostigmine
B intravenous trimetaphan
C intravenous naloxone
D stellate ganglion block
E intramuscular atropine.

II.21 Antibiotics known to interfere with neuromuscular transmission include:

A tobramycin
B cefotaxime
C gentamicin
D amikacin
E metronidazole.

II.22 A left-sided Robertshaw double lumen endobronchial tube:

A can be used for left lower lobectomy
B is suitable for a right-sided bronchopleural fistula
C has its two lumens lying side by side
D is preferable to a right-sided tube wherever possible
E is contra-indicated in a patient with a right pneumothorax.

II.23 In a patient with bilateral bronchiectasis undergoing elective abdominal hysterectomy:

A head-up tilt should be avoided
B endobronchial intubation is required
C awake intubation is indicated
D spontaneous ventilation with epidural anaesthesia is contra-indicated
E preoperative anaemia is a likely finding.

II.24 The following are true of the brachial plexus:

A it is formed from the anterior primary rami of T5–C1
B the lateral cord has contributions from C5–7
C the posterior cord has contributions from C5–T1
D the three cords are related to the first rib and emerge from beneath pectoralis minor
E the median nerve is the continuation of the medial cord.

II.25 The following are true of the nerve supply to the arm:

A tourniquet damage to the radial nerve will result in loss of supination
B traumatic damage to the ulnar nerve at the elbow results in a useless hand
C damage to the median nerve by a superficial wrist laceration that avoids the motor components results in only minor disability
D fracture of the radial head can damage the posterior interosseous branch of the radial nerve
E a supracondylar fracture of the humerus can damage the median nerve.

II.26 The following are factors that aid the competence of the oesophagogastric junction:

A a sling of diaphragmatic smooth muscle
B folds of mucosa
C intra-abdominal pressure tending to close the oesophageal lumen
D the administration of morphine
E the administration of metoclopramide.

II.27 Considering the nerve supply to the anterior abdominal wall:

- **A** the skin over the xiphisternum is supplied by T7
- **B** the skin at the umbilicus is supplied by T10
- **C** the skin in the groin is supplied by L1
- **D** L1 divides into the ilio-inguinal and ilio-epigastric nerves
- **E** the ilio-inguinal nerve does not supply abdominal skin.

II.28 The mandibular division of the trigeminal nerve:

- **A** accompanies the lesser mandibular artery through the foramen ovale
- **B** can be blocked by slipping anteriorly off the lateral pterygoid plate
- **C** has two sensory ganglia, the otic and submandibular, in which the sensory nerves synapse
- **D** supplies sensation to both the inside and outside of the cheek
- **E** supplies sensation to the skin of the temple.

II.29 The sciatic nerve:

- **A** contains the largest nerve fibres in the body
- **B** with the posterior cutaneous nerve of thigh supplies sensation to the back of the leg
- **C** supplies sensation from the lateral side of the foot to the web between the first and second toes
- **D** gives articular fibres to all the joints of the leg
- **E** gives off no major muscular branches between 1–2 cm below the popliteal fossa and a line joining the malleoli.

II.30 Bilateral damage to the recurrent laryngeal nerves:

- **A** causes aphonia
- **B** causes respiratory embarrassment
- **C** causes tetany
- **D** prevents the normal inspiratory abduction of the cords
- **E** allows the vocal cords to assume the cadaveric position.

II.31 Acute intermittent porphyria may present as:

- **A** acute chest pain
- **B** haemoglobinuria
- **C** intra-operative hypotension
- **D** anaemia
- **E** convulsions.

II.32 An increase in plasma potassium to abnormal values causes:

- **A** U-waves on the electrocardiogram
- **B** tall peaked T-waves
- **C** prolonged QRS complexes
- **D** ventricular fibrillation
- **E** an increase in digitalis toxicity.

II.33 In a patient with constrictive pericarditis, likely clinical features include:

A tiredness
B hepatomegaly
C a third heart sound
D a forceful apex beat
E pulsus paradoxus.

II.34 Common complications of acute myocardial infarction include:

A hypertension
B left ventricular failure
C ventriculoseptal defect
D ventricular aneurysm
E sinus bradycardia.

II.35 An opening snap heard on cardiac auscultation:

A is indicative of a fixed rigid AV valve
B is louder during expiration
C is associated with mitral stenosis
D follows the second heart sound
E is best heard at the upper border of the sternum.

II.36 The T-wave on the ECG is:

A representative of repolarization of the ventricles
B less than 2 mV in the standard leads
C increased in amplitude in hyperkalaemia
D increased in amplitude in digitalis toxicity
E normal in atrial fibrillation.

II.37 Causes of systemic hypertension include:

A polycystic renal disease
B Cushing's syndrome
C myxoedema
D subarachnoid haemorrhage
E ischaemic heart disease.

II.38 Concerning adult panhypopituitarism:

A its eponym is Sheehan's disease
B hypoglycaemic episodes occur
C there is adrenal insufficiency
D there is amenorrhoea
E treatment includes mineralocorticoids.

II.39 Raised urinary excretion of 4-hydroxy-, 3-methoxy-mandelic acid (VMA) is commonly found in association with:

A melanoma
B pregnancy
C phaeochromocytoma
D diabetes insipidus
E carcinomatosis.

II.40 Syncope is a recognized feature of the following:

A diabetes mellitus
B aortic stenosis
C haemophilia
D after a bout of coughing
E standing for long periods in hot weather.

II.41 Drugs used in the conservative management of ulcerative colitis include:

A azathioprine
B indomethacin
C prednisolone
D codeine phosphate
E sulphasalazine

II.42 Likely causes of persistent diarrhoea include:

A thyrotoxicosis
B intestinal intussusception
C ulcerative colitis
D food allergy
E hypokalaemia.

II.43 Causes of cirrhosis include:

A viral hepatitis
B haemochromatosis
C cardiomyopathy
D secondary syphilis
E cystic fibrosis.

II.44 Primary haemostasis depends upon:

A blood coagulation
B platelet aggregation and adhesiveness
C vascular factors
D prostaglandin release
E serotonin.

II.45 Neurofibromatosis is associated with:
- A osteomalacia
- B paraplegia
- C phaeochromocytoma
- D aortic stenosis
- E increased incidence of gliomata.

II.46 Myaesthenic syndrome differs from true myaesthenia because:
- A there is increased sensitivity to depolarizing neuromuscular blocking drugs
- B there is decreased EMG voltage
- C there is resistance to non-depolarizing neuromuscular blocking drugs
- D the EMG shows post-tetanic facilitation
- E anticholinesterases are of little benefit.

II.47 Dextran 70:
- A has an average molecular weight lower than albumin
- B can cause acute anaphylaxis
- C is largely cleared from the blood in four hours
- D cannot be mixed with dextrose
- E causes haemodilution and reduces haemoglobin concentration.

II.48 In aspirin overdose:
- A coma is common
- B the patient may complain of tinnitus
- C forced acid diuresis should be considered if the plasma salicylate exceeds 50 mg/100 ml
- D hyperventilation is usual
- E there will always be an acidosis.

II.49 The following would be indications for dialysis:
- A serum potassium of above 5 mmol/l
- B a plasma bicarbonate of 10 mEq/l
- C creatinine clearance of less than 3 ml/min
- D a rise of blood urea of 8 mmol/l/day
- E rate of change of any parameter is more important than the absolute level.

II.50 In pulmonary embolism:
- A serum LDH is normal
- B characteristic ECG changes are S3 Q1
- C warfarin is a suitable first-line anticoagulant
- D high-dose steroids are indicated
- E jaundice only occurs if there is pulmonary infarction.

II.51 The development of pulmonary fibrosis is associated with:

- A hypersensitivity
- B rheumatoid arthritis
- C paraquat poisoning
- D pulmonary embolism
- E uraemia.

II.52 Bilateral hilar lymphadenopathy is a feature of:

- A pulmonary tuberculosis
- B Hodgkin's disease
- C sarcoidosis
- D pneumoconiosis
- E systemic lupus erythematosus.

II.53 Pulmonary oxygen toxicity is associated with, or occurs as a result of:

- A prolonged oxygen therapy
- B high altitude
- C increased metabolic rate
- D raised $PaCO_2$
- E anaemia.

II.54 Acute pancreatitis causes:

- A disseminated intravascular coagulation
- B paralytic ileus
- C hypocalcaemia
- D hypoxia
- E hyperkalaemia.

II.55 Two days following an uncomplicated nephrectomy for hydronephrosis, a 27-year-old woman develops a temperature of 38.1°C. The following are likely causes:

- A absorption of sequestered retroperitoneal blood
- B post-operative chest infection
- C atelectasis
- D pulmonary embolus
- E sub-phrenic abscess.

II.56 The following features are consistent with a diagnosis of acute arterial occlusion of the lower limb:

- A pain
- B paralysis
- C pallor
- D oedema
- E cold.

II.57 The following are true of diverticulitis:

- **A** the sigmoid colon and rectum are most commonly affected
- **B** the incidence increases with age
- **C** there is an increased risk of malignant change
- **D** an acute attack should be treated surgically
- **E** probanthine is a useful drug.

II.58 When a gallstone impacts in a bile duct:

- **A** the gall bladder is usually impalpable
- **B** jaundice is followed by severe, colicky pain
- **C** the urine becomes dark
- **D** an accompanying pyrexia should be treated with tetracycline
- **E** liver function rapidly becomes depressed.

II.59 The following are true of Paget's disease:

- **A** it is a rare disease of disordered bone architecture
- **B** any bone can be affected
- **C** pathological fracture is a fairly common presentation
- **D** sarcomatous change occurs
- **E** surgery is best avoided for osteoarthritis of the hip secondary to the disease.

II.60 The following are true of rupture of the bladder:

- **A** most cases are consequent on urinary retention
- **B** the patient has a painful desire to pass urine
- **C** intravenous pyelography is a useful investigation
- **D** the patient should be catheterized with a small urethral catheter prior to surgery
- **E** the need for surgery is urgent.

Paper II Answers

II.1 **TFTFF**

A Not used commonly now.
B Not an anaesthetic unless given in large enough doses to produce cardiovascular depression.
D Too cardiovascularly depressant.
E Too high an incidence of dysrhythmias.

II.2 **TTTFF**

A similar question to I.3, and a common topic for discussion.

D,E Neither are contra-indications to general anaesthesia — the question does not specify whether this is to be done in a dental surgery or hospital.

II.3 **FTFFF**

A He MUST have a chest X-ray: he may have a co-existing inoperable bronchogenic carcinoma.
B Certainly.
C Justifiable, not mandatory.
D Induction in ventilatory obstruction is a much-asked question: there are a number of approaches; this is not one.
E Not necessarily.

II.4 **TFTFT**

The question asks for those that are NOT compensated.

B These are temperature-compensated, being surrounded by an insulating jacket.
D The E.M.O. contains a compensatory bellows and a temperature range indicator for safe use.

II.5 **TTTTT**

C Often used in the elderly as premedication.
E Rather than hyoscine in the elderly.

II.6 TTFTF

C Not complete until plane 4.
E Gradually diminishes over planes 1,2.

II.7 FTFTT

A This is an ideal recipe for cerebral hypoxia.
C Last resort for failure to VENTILATE, not failure to INTUBATE.

II.8 TTTFT

D Does not affect production, only its conversion to carbonic acid.
E Although profound unconsciousness may reduce CO_2 production to basal levels, many unconscious patients are pyrexial and hyperdynamic.

II.9 TTTFT

D Fibrinolytic activation is responsible for many of the bleeding problems that occur in this condition.

II.10 TFFFF

B Certainly not if this is a single isolated finding: increased inspired oxygen is the first-line treatment.
C,D,E None of these are indications for elective post-operative ventilation.

II.11 FFTFF

A Only if the local anaesthetic spreads to block the recurrent laryngeal nerve.
B Meiosis.
D This is the superior laryngeal nerve.
E Possibly, but intracranial sympathetic supply is relatively unimportant.

II.12 TFTFT

B Controlled ventilation to reduce pCO_2, which by inducing vasconstriction improves picture quality.
D No, may severely reduce cerebral blood flow.
E Because of the likelihood of carotid sinus stimulation.

II.13 TTFFT

This is acute section of the spinal cord, with interruption of the sympathetic supply.

C The patient should not be given suxamethonium because of potassium release, but there is no change in sensitivity to the drug.
D Vasodilation will produce cooling and hypothermia.

II.14 FFFTT

A,B,C We are talking about the pregnant uterus and none of these significantly reduces uterine tone.

II.15 FFTFF

A,B Although in some cases epidurals may be avoided in these situations, the contra-indications to their use would only be relative.
D Epidurals are often used to facilitate assisted delivery.
E Epidurals are specifically used to reduce hypertension.

II.16 TTFTT

C The reservoir tube is to prevent dilution of inspired gas by room air, not to prevent rebreathing.

II.17 TFTFT

A,C Neither of these presents frequent problems unless systemic absorption of excessively large amounts of opioid occurs.

II.18 TTTFT

D Anaesthetic concentrations build up more quickly in closed systems.

II.19 TTFFT

C Although some barbiturates are specific enzyme inducers, thiopentone is not long-acting enough to do this.

D No analgesic properties.

II.20 FTFTF

A Little effect, but constriction if anything.

C Naloxone will reverse pupillary constriction induced by opiates, otherwise it has no effect on the pupils.

E Intramuscular atropine in normal dosage has little, if any, effect.

II.21 TFTTF

B,E Neither are aminoglycosides and have not been implicated.

II.22 TTTTF

A The tube is no further distal than the main bronchus.
E May well be indicated if artificial ventilation is essential.

II.23 TFFFT

B Not for elective hysterectomy.
C Not necessary
D Satisfactory as long as patient is positioned head-down, though coughing may be a problem.

II.24 TTTFF

D The three trunks form the six divisions at the lateral border of the first rib; the cords are more distal.
E The median has contributions from the lateral and medial cords; the ulnar is the continuation of the medial cord.

II.25 FFFTT

A Supination in flexion is biceps (musculocutaneous).
B Trick movements can compensate.
C Loss of palmar sensation is a major disability.
D This is a motor branch.

II.26 FTTFT

A True — but the diaphragm is striated muscle.
C Under normal circumstances this is true; too high a pressure will reduce competence.
D There is no true sphincter here for morphine to constrict. It also causes gastric atony and is an emetic.

II.27 TTTFT

D This is a bit of a trick question, unlikely to occur in the actual exam and included here to draw attention to the advice to READ THE QUESTION: not ilioEPIgastric but ilioHYPOgastric.

E True: it goes through the inguinal ring to supply skin over the inner thigh and part of the genitalia.

II.28 FFFTT

A Through the foramen ovale — but the artery is a red herring. A branch, the nervus spinosus, goes through the foramen spinosus with the middle meningeal artery to supply sensation to part of the dura.

B Posteriorly off the plate.

C Ganglia, yes, but no sensory, only parasympathetic, synapses.

E Shared with the zygomatic branch of the ophthalmic division.

II.29 FTFTF

A It is the largest nerve, but the fibres in it have the same range of diameters as in any other mixed nerve.

C Its branches supply the entire foot except for a variable area between the medial malleolus and the base of the great toe (saphenous from femoral).

II.30 FTFTF

A Causes dysphonia and dyspnoea, but not aphonia.

C Tetany would only be caused by hypocapnoea. The ASSOCIATION would be parathyroid surgery, but that is not CAUSATION.

E The cords remain adducted by the cricothyroid muscles (superior laryngeal nerve).

II.31 FFFFT

A The likely association is with acute abdominal pain.

B It is the abnormal porphyrins, rather than haemoglobin, which colour the urine.

C If anything, there can be hypertension.

D Not normally associated.

E May present as epileptiform convulsions.

II.32 FTTTT

Hyperkalaemia also causes AV conduction defects and reduced amplitude of the P-waves.

II.33 TTTFT

D The apex beat will be remote and hard to feel.
E Does occur, together with a rapid, low-volume pulse (was asked in I.37E).

II.34 TTFFT

A Either hypotension or hypertension can be complication of an acute myocardial infarction.
C,D Although these are documented complications, they are NOT COMMON.

II.35 FTTTF

A Indicates a mobile rather than a fixed valve.
E Is maximal just inside the apex of the heart.

II.36 TTTFT

B A generous margin! It is usually far less than 1 mV.
C Asked in II.32B.
D The ST segment shows the 'reverse-tick' in digitalis therapy. The onset of toxicity is not reflected in any specific way in the ECG.

II.37 TTFTF

C Hypotension if anything.
E May be associated with, but it is not a cause.

II.38 FTTTF

A Its eponym is Simmond's disease. Sheehan's syndrome is hypopituitarism caused by infarction secondary to haemorrhage in labour.
E Glucocorticoids yes, not mineralocorticoids.

II.39 FFTFF

A,B,D,E VMA is a catecholamine metabolite and is not COMMONLY associated with any of these conditions.

II.40 TTFTT

Syncope occurs in these conditions because of:

A autonomic neuropathy;
B fixed cardiac output;
C there is no special reason why haemophiliacs should faint;
D failure of venous return;
E peripheral vasodilatation and pooling.

II.41 TFTTT

B Indomethacin is a non-steroidal anti-inflammatory drug that tends to cause bowel ulceration.

II.42 TFTFF

B Intussusception is not associated with persistent diarrhoea and may produce obstruction.
D The key word is persistent: allergy will cause acute diarrhoea.
E Hypokalaemia causes constipation.

II.43 TTTFT

D Congenital, but not secondary syphilis.

II.44 FTTTF

A Coagulation is a secondary effect.
D Platelet contact releases prostaglandin endoperoxidase and thromboxane, both of which alter platelet shape.
E Not primary haemostasis.

II.45 **TTTTT**

A–E Neurofibromata may develop in many sites, causing all these.

II.46 **FTFTT**

A,C In myaesthenic syndrome, there may be even more sensitivity to non-depolarizers than in true myaesthenia: there is no difference in response to depolarizers.

II.47 **FTFFT**

A Molecular weight of albumin is 67 000.
C Much longer — 12–16 hours.
D Is presented in 5% dextrose or 0.9% saline.

II.48 **FTFTF**

A Only in children.
C The level is correct, but it is a forced alkaline diuresis: alkali is given to speed excretion of the acid.
E Not necessarily, and it depends at what stage the acid-base state is checked. Aspirin has very complex effects on acid-base balance.

II.49 **FTFTT**

A 6–7 mmol/l K^+.
B 10–15 mmol/l bicarbonate.

II.50 **FFFFT**

A Raised.
B S1, Q3, T3.
C No, initial heparinization and only long-term warfarin.
D No good evidence.

II.51 TTTTT

A E.g. Farmer's, bird-fancier's lung, etc.
D Multiple pulmonary infarcts following embolism.

II.52 FTTFF

A Not bilateral — tuberculosis tends to be unilateral.
D Diffuse lung lesions are diagnostic of pneumoconiosis, not lymphadenopathy.
E Hilar lymphadenopathy is not a diagnostic feature of SLE.

II.53 TFFFF

B Oxygen partial pressures are reduced, not elevated, at altitude.
C,D,E Oxygen toxicity is a direct effect of oxygen on the lungs.

II.54 TTTTF

E Usually hypokalaemia following persistent vomiting and associated bowel disturbances.

II.55 FFTFF

A There won't be much blood retroperitoneally after an uncomplicated nephrectomy.
B,D,E 2 days is too early for a chest infection, abscess or pulmonary embolus.

II.56 TTTFT

Pain and pallor are the earliest symptoms of acute occlusion; the limb will not take long to become cold. Paralysis takes a little longer to develop as nerve conduction fails.

D Hydrostatic pressure in the limb is low, preventing oedema formation (a sign of venous occlusion).

II.57 FTFFT

A The sigmoid colon is affected in the majority of cases. The rectum is not affected.

C Diverticular disease is not pre-malignant; however, it is important not to miss a co-existing cancer.

D,E Treat medically unless unbearable or complications develop (e.g. bleeding, fistulae). Probanthine is an antispasmodic.

II.58 TFTFF

B Pain usually occurs first (and often suddenly).

D Tetracycline is reasonable for acute cholecystitis, but jaundice plus accompanying pyrexia equals urgent operation.

E Serum liver enzymes will soon become abnormal, but function will not become depressed for some time.

II.59 FTTTT

A Paget's disease is common.

E Surgery is hazardous because the bone is very hard and abnormally vascular.

II.60 FFTFT

A The majority are secondary to trauma. A full bladder is more likely to rupture after a direct blow.

Paper III Questions

III.1 During surgery for insertion of a permanent indwelling pacemaker:

A ventricular fibrillation may occur at any stage
B the use of muscle relaxants is contra-indicated
C atropine is contra-indicated
D halothane should not be used
C a temporary pacemaker should have been inserted preoperatively.

III.2 Likely complications of chair dental anaesthesia in the supine position include:

A regurgitation
B postural hypotension
C aspiration
D cardiac arrhythmias
E hypoglycaemia.

III.3 The following are suitable techniques for hypotensive anaesthesia for major head and neck surgery:

A intravenous increments of phentolamine
B d-tubocurarine and halothane
C intravenous phenoxybenzamine at induction
D an intradural injection of 3.5 ml of 0.5% heavy bupivacaine
E an infusion of sodium nitroprusside.

III.4 Vaporisers suitable for use in a draw-over mode include:

A Fluotec mark 4
B Oxford miniature vaporiser (OMV)
C E.M.O.
D Goldman
E copper kettle.

III.5 The use of nitrous oxide anaesthesia may be contra-indicated in patients presenting with or for:

A air embolism
B intestinal obstruction and bowel distension
C pneumothorax
D middle-ear surgery
E air encephalography.

III.6 Concerning eye signs of anaesthesia:

A the eyelash reflex disappears in stage 2
B the corneal reflex is absent throughout stage 3
C by plane 2 of stage 3, the pupils are small and eye movements have ceased
D the pupillary light reflex is abolished in plane 3, stage 3
E oculomotor paralysis, in stage 4, produces mydriasis.

III.7 Four hours after general anaesthesia for elective cholecystectomy, a patient is breathless and distressed with a mild tachycardia and a blood pressure of 170/100. Blood gases show PaO_2 9 kPa (70 mm Hg), $PaCO_2$ 9 kPa (70 mm Hg) and a bicarbonate of 28 mmol/l. Likely diagnoses include:

A pulmonary segmental collapse
B blood loss
C metabolic acidosis
D over-transfusion
E hypoventilation.

III.8 Genetic factors likely to influence elective general anaesthesia include:

A porphyria
B malignant hyperpyrexia
C atypical pseudocholinesterase
D sickle-cell disease
E glucose-6-phosphate dehydrogenase deficiency.

III.9 Patients at greater than normal risk of developing gram-negative septicaemia include those suffering from:

A diabetes mellitus
B cirrhosis
C leukaemia
D polycythaemia
E uraemia.

III.10 A fit person, who has been hit by a car, comes into hospital with a compound fracture of the tibia. There is no other obvious injury. Following correction of the fracture under uncomplicated general anaesthesia, the patient fails to regain consciousness as expected, despite good general condition. Serious consideration should now be given to:

A subdural haematoma
B cerebral fat embolism
C bilateral pneumothorax
D hypovolaemia requiring blood replacement
E massive pulmonary embolism.

III.11 Common approaches to apply local anaesthetic to the brachial plexus include:

- **A** axillary
- **B** interscalene
- **C** infraclavicular
- **D** subclavian
- **E** supraclavicular.

III.12 During pneumoencephalography:

- **A** cardiac dysrhythmias are a common problem
- **B** neuroleptanaesthesia is the technique of choice
- **C** apnoea may occur
- **D** nitrous oxide is contra-indicated
- **E** vomiting on recovery is a common problem.

III.13 Epidural anaesthesia in labour:

- **A** is contra-indicated in patients with sickle-cell disease
- **B** masks placental abruption
- **C** increases placental blood flow
- **D** masks uterine rupture
- **E** is contra-indicated in patients with peripheral neuropathy.

III.14 In the Apgar scoring system of neonatal asphyxia:

- **A** a weak cry or hypoventilation scores 1
- **B** blue hands or feet score 1
- **C** absent reflex responses scores 0
- **D** a heart rate in excess of 80 scores 2
- **E** a single assessment at 1 minute will distinguish between primary and terminal apnoea.

III.15 Techniques of analgesia approved by the Central Midwives Board for use by midwives include:

- **A** continuous flow Entonox®
- **B** trichloroethylene inhaler (Emotril)®
- **C** trichloroethylene inhaler (Tecota)®
- **D** institution and maintenance of epidural local anaesthesia through an indwelling catheter
- **E** intramuscular pethidine.

III.16 The following cause respiratory problems in the neonate:

- **A** choanal atresia
- **B** Pierre-Robin syndrome
- **C** laryngomalacia
- **D** Treacher-Collins syndrome
- **E** Eaton-Lambert syndrome.

III.17 Suitable alternative methods for the relief of post-operative pain following elective cholecystectomy include:

A cryoanalgesia
B transcutaneous nerve stimulation
C epidural chlorocresol
D subcutaneous infusion of opiate
E sustained release morphine.

III.18 Anticholinergic premedication:

A helps prevent regurgitation
B reduces postoperative nausea and vomiting caused by opiates
C produces a rise in body temperature
D causes arterial hypoxaemia
E interferes with pupillary responses under anaesthesia.

III.19 Etomidate is:

A contra-indicated in atopic patients
B rapidly metabolized in the liver
C diabetogenic
D suitable for use in patients with acute intermittent porphyria
E suitable for use in patients with raised intracranial pressure.

III.20 In a patient receiving monoamineoxidase inhibitor therapy and presenting for elective cholecystectomy, anaesthetic management should include:

A the avoidance of morphine premedication
B postponement of surgery for 1 week
C subcutaneous heparin
D preoperative beta-adrenergic blockade
E anticholinergic premedication.

III.21 Postoperative hepatic failure has been associated with the use of:

A halothane
B methoxyflurane
C trichloroethylene
D nitrous oxide
E isoflurane.

III.22 During one-lung anaesthesia:

A perfusion to the dependent lung increases
B ventilation to the dependent lung is reduced
C ventilation/perfusion mismatching is more marked before the diseased lung is collapsed than after
D anatomical dead space is reduced
E pulmonary vascular resistance is reduced.

III.23 A 3-year-old child presents in the accident department, thought to have inhaled a peanut 2 hours previously. A reasonable scheme of anaesthetic management for bronchoscopy and removal of the foreign body would include:

A premedication with atropine
B gaseous induction with halothane
C the avoidance of nitrous oxide
D emergence anaesthetic technique
E bronchopulmonary lavage.

III.24 The following are true of the cervical plexus:

A it is formed from the anterior rami of all the cervical nerves
B there are, in general, four groups of branches of each ramus
C it supplies motor fibres to the phrenic nerve, the largest contribution being from C4
D branches from C1–3 form the great auricular nerve which has auricular, facial and mastoid branches
E branches from C2–3 form the anterior cutaneous nerve of the neck.

III.25 The brachial artery:

A is readily palpable throughout its length
B is crossed by the bicipital aponeurosis
C is crossed by the medial cubital vein
D is crossed from lateral to medial by the median nerve
E divides at the wrist into the ulnar and radial arteries.

III.26 The following are true of the diaphragm:

A its complex development includes a muscular contribution from the cervical region
B its sensory nerves all come from the vagus and cervical sympathetic chain
C posteriorly it forms the arcuate ligaments that insert into psoas major and quadratus lumborum
D it is the most resistant striated muscle to non-depolarizing neuromuscular blocking agents
E its venous drainage is directly into the inferior vena cava.

III.27 Nerves, remote from the site of operation, likely to be damaged inadvertantly during surgery include:

A median
B saphenous
C facial
D trigeminal
E lateral popliteal.

III.28 The mandibular division of the trigeminal nerve:

A subserves sensation to the anterior third of the tongue and to the floor of the mouth
B subserves cutaneous sensation approximately anterior to a line from the angle of the jaw, through the external auditory meatus, to the vertex
C is the only division with a true motor component
D carries salivary secretomotor fibres
E the lingual nerve and inferior dental nerve are two of its branches.

III.29 Damage to the sciatic nerve by a misplaced intramuscular injection into the buttock:

A can be avoided by using blunt needles
B can be avoided if the injection is given anterior to a line joining the posterior superior iliac spine to the greater trochanter
C can give pressure sores in thin subjects because of anaesthesia over the ischial tuberosity
D will cause weakness or paralysis of all muscles below the knee
E can result in trophic ulcers on the sole of the foot.

III.30 The skin over the occiput and the back of the neck is supplied by:

A a branch from the first cervical nerve
B the medial branch of the second cervical nerve
C the greater occipital nerve
D overlap from the lesser occipital nerve
E the medial and lateral branches of C3–6.

III.31 Hypernatraemia occurs:

A following severe burns
B after intravenous feeding with 50% dextrose
C in hyperaldosteronism
D in renal failure
E in cystic fibrosis.

III.32 Which of the following statements are true?

A a low PaO_2 and $PaCO_2$ are found in interstitial pulmonary fibrosis
B the normal pulmonary vascular resistance is 0–8 units
C a pulmonary artery pressure of 36/21 is within normal limits
D the normal left atrial pressure is less than 5 cm water
E a slow 'y' descent in the jugular waveform is characteristic of tricuspid stenosis.

III.33 Likely causes of cardiomegaly observed on an A-P chest radiograph include:

A congestive cardiac failure
B pleural effusion
C mitral stenosis
D complete heart block
E the normal variation in heart size.

III.34 Causes of pulmonary hypertension include:

A atrioseptal defect
B chronic bronchitis
C pulmonary embolism
D sodium nitroprusside infusion
E high altitude.

III.35 A midsystolic ejection murmur is heard when there is:

A aortic stenosis
B systemic hypertension
C coarctation of the aorta
D atrioseptal defect
E mitral regurgitation.

III.36 Methods commonly used in the detection of venous thrombosis include:

A venography
B Doppler ultrasound
C the use of radioactivity-labelled albumin
D impedance plethysmography
E labelled fibrinogen uptake.

III.37 The jugular venous pulse does not show an 'a' wave in:

A atrial fibrillation
B first-degree heart block
C ventricular tachycardia
D atrial flutter
E pulmonary embolus.

III.38 A 37- year-old diabetic taking 10 U Actrapid® and 18 U Monotard® twice daily presents for major abdominal surgery. The following would be suitable peri-operative regimens to keep his diabetes satisfactorily under control:

A a 10% dextrose infusion containing Actrapid® insulin and potassium
B a depot injection of an ultra-long-acting insulin
C continue his normal injections and start intravenous feeding
D withhold insulin unless his blood sugar rises above 7 mmol/l
E give soluble insulin on a timed sliding scale.

III.39 Hyperthyroidism is likely in a patient presenting for elective thyroidectomy if:

A the patient is febrile
B the heart rate is greater than 100 beats/min
C the patient suffers from stridor
D signs of right heart failure are present
E Chvostek's sign is positive.

III.40 A 17-year-old boy is admitted comatose. He is flushed, pyrexial and shows signs of cerebral irritability. The following are true:

A his trachea should be intubated if he has no gag reflex
B a lumbar puncture could give the diagnosis
C an estimation of the blood sugar is mandatory
D a radiograph of the skull should be obtained
E the signs are consistent with aspirin poisoning.

III.41 Indications for urgent surgical treatment of ulcerative colitis include:

A anaemia
B acute toxic dilation
C development of pyoderma gangrenosa
D to avoid the use of steroids
E severe dehydration caused by intractable diarrhoea.

III.42 Likely causes of persistent dysphagia include:

A Plummer-Vinson syndrome
B pharyngeal pouch
C pseudobulbar palsy
D bronchogenic carcinoma
E oesophageal foreign body.

III.43 Which of the following statements are true of jaundice?

A urinary bilirubin is increased in obstructive jaundice
B urinary urobilinogen is decreased in hepatocellular jaundice
C haemolytic jaundice is associated with a normal urinary urobilinogen
D hepatocellular jaundice results in reduced urinary bilirubin
E faecal stercobilinogen is raised in haemolytic jaundice.

III.44 Vitamin K is used to treat excessive bleeding associated with:

A haemophilia
B scurvy
C heparin overdosage
D oral anticoagulant overdosage
E factor XII deficiency.

III.45 In familial periodic paralysis:

A attacks frequently occur during sleep
B serum potassium is elevated during attacks
C high carbohydrate diet can precipitate an attack
D attacks may be induced by the administration of glucose
E patients are abnormally sensitive to depolarizing neuromuscular blocking drugs.

III.46 A headache is likely not to be of organic origin if:

A it is aggravated by straining at stool
B the presentation is of mental depression
C the headache is unremitting and not localized
D it is worse in the morning
E skull radiography and CAT scan (tomography) are normal.

III.47 Pharmacological effects of nicotine include:

A hypotension
B vasodilation
C antidiuretic hormone release
D autonomic ganglionic depression
E respiratory stimulation.

III.48 Infusion with dextran solutions cause:

A decreased coagulability
B antigen reactions
C difficulties with cross-matching of blood type
D damage to renal tubules
E rouleaux formation of red blood cells.

III.49 Acute renal failure:

A follows severe hypovolaemia
B the urine SG will be 1010
C frusemide 1–2 g i.v. can be given in the early stages
D potassium must be given to maintain the plasma potassium level
E an intravenous pyelogram is a useless investigation.

III.50 In chronic respiratory acidosis with renal compensation:

A the pH is reduced
B $PaCO_2$ is elevated
C base excess increases
D standard bicarbonate is reduced
E blood CO_2 content is reduced.

III.51 The following are important in the aetiology of a lung abscess:

A pharyngeal pouch
B staphylococcal pneumonia
C septicaemia
D bronchopleural fistula
E pulmonary embolism.

III.52 A reduced FEV_1/FVC ratio is found:

A in restrictive lung disease
B in obstructive lung disease
C when the static compliance is decreased
D in children
E in fibrosing alveolitis.

III.53 Common presenting symptoms of primary bronchogenic carcinoma include:

A finger clubbing
B peripheral neuropathy
C coin shadow on chest radiograph
D palmar erythema
E Horner's syndrome.

III.54 Factors in the development of acute pancreatitis include:

A haemochromatosis
A previous gastrectomy
C uraemia
D halothane anaesthesia
E hypocalcaemia.

III.55 Ascites:

- **A** will not be present clinically with less than about 500 ml of fluid
- **B** is most commonly caused by congestive cardiac failure
- **C** is a poor prognostic sign in cirrhosis
- **D** should be treated initially with diuretics
- **E** should not be tapped for therapeutic reasons if caused by malignancy.

III.56 The characteristic pain of a duodenal ulcer is:

- **A** periodic, with pain-free periods of several weeks
- **B** associated with vomiting
- **C** worse at night
- **D** exacerbated by smoking
- **E** associated with weight loss.

III.57 Oesophageal varices are associated with:

- **A** achalasia of the cardia
- **B** carcinoma of the oesophagus
- **C** hepatic cirrhosis
- **D** portal venous thrombosis
- **E** chronic pancreatitis.

III.58 The following are true of carcinoma of the rectum:

- **A** blood-borne metastasis occurs late
- **B** the adrenal gland is a not uncommon site of secondaries
- **C** bleeding is the commonest earliest symptom
- **D** pain is an early symptom
- **E** ascites indicates hepatic involvement.

III.59 The following factors would tend to delay union following fracture of a long bone:

- **A** malnutrition
- **B** a fracture in a child less than 9 months old
- **C** the site of the fracture
- **D** pathological fracture
- **E** a fracture in a patient more than 60 years old.

III.60 Post-operative retention of urine:

- **A** is particularly common after haemorrhoidectomy
- **B** is likely to follow spinal anaesthesia
- **C** is commoner in men
- **D** may be treated initially with a single dose of frusemide
- **E** is frequently painless.

Paper III Answers

III.1 **TFFFF**

B,C,D None are contra-indicated in normal patients.

E Although a number of patients will have a temporary pacemaker in situ, it is not an essential prerequisite to operation.

III.2 **TFTTF**

B Not a likely complication of the supine position.

E Unlikely to occur except in diabetics.

III.3 **TTFFT**

C A long-acting alpha-adrenergic antagonist.

D This would drop the blood pressure, but is not a sensible approach when you consider the site of operation.

III.4 **FTTTF**

A,E Draw-over vaporisers must be low-resistance; these are not, and are only suitable for plenum use.

III.5 **TTTTT**

A,B,C,D,E All are at risk from the expansion of closed air spaces by the diffusion of nitrous oxide into them down a tension gradient during equilibration with the anaesthetic.

III.6 TFTTF

A Not absent until plane 2.
E Mydriasis in stage 4 is due to deep CNS depression and hypoxia rather than to oculomotor paralysis — that occurs in stage 3, plane 2.

III.7 TFFFT

A,E The cause must be primarily respiratory, due to hypoventilation and probable collapse.
B,D Neither would cause a $PaCO_2$ of 70 mm Hg.
C The bicarbonate of 28 mmol/l excludes this.

III.8 TTTTT

A Mendelian dominant.
B Autosomal dominant but penetrance is incomplete and generations may escape.
C,D Both are recessive genes.
E Sex-linked recessive.

III.9 TTTFT

D Not greater than normal.

III.10 TTFFF

C,D,E The key words are 'despite good general condition'. Thus none of these alternatives can apply.

III.11 TTFFT

C,D Although the infraclavicular approach has been described, the word 'commonly' is in the question.

III.12 TTTTT

A Air in the region of the fourth ventricle often induces cardio-respiratory disorders.

B Suitable because of difficulty in repeatedly moving patients; and spontaneous respiration is used to help show the development of severe respiratory problems.

III.13 FTTTT

A Not contra-indicated unless it impairs respiration!

B,D Arguable, but the safe answer.

III.14 TTTFF

D In excess of 100 is the cut-off point.

E No single assessment will do this. Primary apnoea at one minute will often recover spontaneously, while terminal apnoea will require treatment.

III.15 FTTFT

A Entonox® is certainly approved, but only with a demand flow apparatus held to the face by the patient.

D Midwives are only allowed to top up epidural anaesthetics in which the initial dose has been given by an anaesthetist.

III.16 TTTTF

A–D All are associated with congenital abnormalities of the upper airways.

E This is the myasthenic syndrome associated with a primary bronchogenic carcinoma.

III.17 TTFTF

A Particularly useful in the subcostal or other unilateral incision.
C Chlorocresol, a common preservative in drug ampoules, is a neurolytic agent and can produce a permanent neurological deficit.
D This is a method of systemic administration, not a local application to the wound.
E Oral therapy is unsuitable for post-operative gastro-intestinal surgery.

III.18 FTTTF

A If anything, increased risk of regurgitation.
E Not in normal doses.

III.19 FTFTT

A No reason why, since anaphylaxis is rare.
C No evidence.

III.20 TFFFT

The important word here is ELECTIVE cholecystectomy.
B Postponement must be for at least 2 weeks.
C,D Neither is specifically indicated, the correct treatment being to postpone rather than to try to prevent symptoms.

III.21 TTTFF

A,B,C Here the question does not specify 'commonly', 'likely', etc., and so anything goes, however rare: nitrous oxide and isoflurane have not been implicated (yet!).

III.22 TFTTF

B Ventilation must at least remain the same, but usually increases, especially if the patient is being artificially ventilated.

E Will rise acutely as the other lung is devascularized.

III.23 TTFTF

A No real contra-indication to the use of a drying agent, and indicated if an emergence technique with halothane is to be used.

C Not unless a large area of air trapping occurs distal to the obstruction.

D Children wake up relatively quickly from inhalational anaesthesia, and it is reassuring to have a skilled operator doing the brochoscopy when using an emergence technique.

E Not used.

III.24 FTTFF

A C1–4.

B Communicating, superficial, deep and phrenic.

D True — but C2–3 only; C1 is motor only.

III.25 TTFTF

B,C The aponeurosis lies between the median cubital vein and the brachial artery.

E It divides just below the elbow joint.

III.26 TFTTF

A Motor supply is (mostly) from the phrenic nerve (C3–5).

B There is a somatic sensory supply from the lower thoracic segments.

D It is relatively resistant to depolarizing agents as well.

III.27 FTFFT

A The words 'likely' and 'during operation' make this option false, although damage from inadvertent injection has been reported.
B At the medial malleolus.
C,D Neither is likely to be damaged, though branches might be.
E At the neck of the fibula.

III.28 FTTTT

A Anterior two-thirds of tongue. You could argue that, as it carries sensation to two-thirds, it must carry sensation to one-third — but we would suggest that it is not sensible to encourage semantic arguments!
D Originally from the facial nerve via the chorda tympani.

III.29 FTFTT

A Think before you answer!
C Supplied by posterior primary rami.
D And the hamstrings.

III.30 FTTTF

The general pattern of afferent innervation is from the medial branches of the posterior primary rami; the lateral branches (**E**) are normally motor. C1 is motor only.

C C2: the largest posterior primary ramus.
D There is overlap anteriorly with this branch of the anterior primary ramus (via the cervical plexus).
E C3–5 supply the posterior skin; C6–8 do not.

III.31 TTTTF

B Water is needed to excrete the glucose.
D Renal failure can cause polyuria.
E Sweat sodium is high, not serum sodium.

III.32 TFFFT

C Normal is 25/10.
D Normal is around 12 cm water.

III.33 TFTTT

B A pericardial, but not a pleural, effusion will increase heart size.
D Due to increased ventricular size.
E Heart size can only be assessed accurately on a P-A film.

III.34 TTTFT

A Hyperdynamic circulation.
B,E Vasoconstriction secondary to hypoxia.
D SNP lowers pulmonary and systemic blood pressure.

III.35 TTFTF

C Coarctation produces a late systolic murmur, extending into the second heart sound.
E Mitral regurgitation produces a pansystolic murmur.

III.36 TTFFT

The question includes the word 'commonly'.
C,D Both have been used, but are not common methods.

III.37 TFFTF

The 'a' wave reflects venous distension caused by right atrial contraction and is therefore absent in (**A**) and (**D**). There is an increased delay before the carotid pulse in (**B**). 'a' waves will occur in (**C**) (some, when the tricuspid valve is closed, will be exaggerated) but will not be easy to see. Any obstruction to right ventricular emptying (**E**) would tend to exaggerate them.

III.38 TFFFT

A,E Both are effective: the continuous infusion is in favour at the moment as the mode of most sensitive control.

B,C There is no place for long-acting insulins in the peri-operative period. There is no indication for intravenous feeding.

D Most authorities think that one should never withhold insulin totally.

III.39 TTFTF

C Stridor is caused by thyroid enlargement, but it is not necessarily a feature of hyperthyroidism.

E A positive Chvostek's sign is a sign of low serum ionized calcium that may be found in hypoparathyroidism.

III.40 FTTFF

A The requirement would be to nurse him semi-prone.

B He could have meningitis or encephalitis.

C Easy to do and a sensible precaution in any undiagnosed coma.

D Not unless there is a history of head injury.

E Coma is rare except in children. It can cause convulsions, but why should he be flushed and pyrexial?

III.41 FTTFF

A Anaemia is not an indication for urgent surgery in ulcerative colitis.

D This is not a surgical indication.

E This must be treated urgently before anaesthesia and surgery are considered safe.

III.42 TTTTF

A Oesophageal web.

D By compression.

E Dysphagia won't be persistent.

III.43 TFFFT

Know your jaundices!

B Normal or increased unless there is obstruction.

C Urinary urobilinogen is increased in haemolytic jaundice.

D Hepatocellular jaundice results in normal or increased urinary bilirubin.

III.44 FFFTF

A Factor VIII is not vitamin-K-dependent.

B Vitamin C deficiency leading to capillary fragility.

C Heparin does not affect prothrombin.

E Factor XII is not prothrombin-dependent.

III.45 TFTTF

B Normal or hypokalaemia.

E Normal response to succinylcholine.

III.46 FFTFF

Note the stem says, '. . . NOT . . . of organic origin'.

A,D Both are signs of raised intracranial pressure.

B Depressed patients get headaches, but frontal lobe tumours in particular present with mental change.

C The classical psychoneurotic headache, but a dangerous diagnosis to make hastily.

E There are many organic causes in which both tests would be entirely normal.

III.47 FFTTT

A,B Cutaneous vasoconstriction, tachycardia and hypertension.

C Transient stimulation followed by depression.

III.48 TTTTF

A Reduces platelet aggregation, destabilizes fibrin and activates plasmin.

D Dextran 40 can cause acute renal failure.

E Dextrans reduce rouleaux formation.

III.49 TFTFF

B Urinary SG may be 1010 but not necessarily: there may be no urine at all.

C It is arguable whether frusemide can actually halt the development of acute renal failure, but many would advocate its use.

E An intravenous pyelogram may show a nephrogram and can be useful in diagnosis.

III.50 TTTFF

A Compensation is never complete, so the pH will still be lower than normal.

D In a chronic acidosis, with renal compensation the bicarbonate is usually elevated.

E Blood CO_2 content will be raised.

III.51 TTTTF

A Encourages aspiration.

C Septic emboli.

E Not unless associated with sepsis.

III.52 FTFFF

A Both FEV_1 and FVC are reduced: (**E**) is an example.

C Resistance, not compliance, affects the ratio.

III.53 TTTFT

The inclusion of 'common' is difficult.

B,E Possibly not common enough! — Horner's occurs because of involvement of the cervical sympathetics.

III.54 TTTFF

D Hepatic, but not pancreatic disease.

E An effect, not a cause. Hypercalcaemia is a cause.

III.55 TTFFF

C Ascites may be present for years in stable cirrhotics.

D Diuretics are indicated when the ascites is caused by congestive cardiac failure. They are sometimes helpful in other cases.

E There is the danger of seeding but, if indicated, relief of the patient's discomfort overrides that.

III.56 TFTTF

B,E Vomiting and weight loss are characteristic of gastric ulcer.

III.57 FFTTF

A,B Not directly associated with portal hypertension and varices.

E Chronic pancreatitis is associated with alcoholism and cirrhosis but not directly with varices.

III.58 TTTFF

B,D Liver and lungs are the commonest site of secondaries from rectal carcinoma. Pain is usually a late symptom.

E Ascites may be because of liver involvement, but peritoneal seedlings are more likely.

III.59 TFTTF

There is unlikely to be much general orthopaedics in the examination, but an understanding of the basic principles would be expected in an anaesthetist anaesthetizing for orthopaedic surgery.

B,E Young children heal quickly; once adult, age has little effect on union.

III.60 TTTFF

D There is not failure to produce urine, but failure to pass it.

E Patients are commonly in pain and very restless.

Paper IV Questions

IV.1 Appropriate agents for use during synchronized electrical reversal of atrial arrhythmias include:

- **A** diazepam
- **B** midazolam
- **C** etomidate
- **D** thiopentone
- **E** methohexitone.

IV.2 Drugs which can safely be used when anaesthetizing a patient with malignant hyperpyrexia include:

- **A** fentanyl
- **B** atropine
- **C** droperidol
- **D** nitrous oxide
- **E** thiopentone.

IV.3 Indications for general anaesthesia for oral surgery include:

- **A** mental retardation
- **B** local infection
- **C** porphyria
- **D** pregnancy
- **E** ischaemic heart disease.

IV.4 During induction of anaesthesia in a patient with a dental abscess:

- **A** the patient must be preoxygenated
- **B** suxamethonium will provide optimal intubating conditions
- **C** thiopentone is contra-indicated
- **D** blind nasal intubation is contra-indicated
- **E** cricoid pressure should be used to minimize regurgitation.

IV.5 Concerning the sterilization of anaesthetic equipment:

- **A** boiling in water for 15 minutes at atmospheric pressure kills bacteria and spores
- **B** an autoclave pressure of 1 Bar at a temperature of 120° C for 15 minutes will kill all living organisms
- **C** ethylene oxide is only bactericidal
- **D** ethylene oxide takes 2–4 hours to be completely effective
- **E** a 0.1% solution of chlorhexidine will sterilize an endotracheal tube in 3 minutes.

IV.6 During anaesthesia in a susceptible patient, the following are known to precipitate a sickle-cell crisis:

A hypoxia
B hypercarbia
C hypotension
D alkalosis
E hypothermia.

IV.7 Concerning the abolition of reflex activity during anaesthesia:

A the gag reflex is abolished in plane 2, stage 3
B carinal stimulation will induce coughing during surgical anaesthesia above stage 4
C anal dilation will produce laryngospasm in stage 3
D traction on the external ocular muscles commonly produces tachycardia
E tracheal tug is often seen with intercostal paralysis.

IV.8 Factors associated with the development of post-operative pulmonary collapse include:

A atropine premedication
B emphysema
C ankylosing spondylitis
D urinary retention
E spinal anaesthesia.

IV.9 Peri-operative haemorrhage in a haemophiliac undergoing emergency surgery can be satisfactorily treated with:

A transfusion of fresh whole blood
B transfusion of plasma
C human AHG
D epsilon-aminocaproic acid
E porcine AHG.

IV.10 Measures commonly used in the treatment of gram-negative septicaemia include:

A beta-adrenergic blockade
B the transfusion of fresh frozen plasma
C the infusion of 8.4% sodium bicarbonate
D alpha-adrenergic blockade
E intravenous heparin.

IV.11 In the casualty department, a 45-year-old man falls to the ground. You can feel no pulse. You should immediately:
A give mouth-to-mouth resuscitation
B give external cardiac massage
C defibrillate the patient's heart
D inject intracardiac adrenaline
E await recovery from a vaso-vagal attack.

IV.12 Opioid drugs are contra-indicated in neurosurgical patients post-operatively because they:
A produce respiratory depression
B produce mydriasis
C depress the cough reflex
D cross the blood–brain barrier
E mask neurological signs.

IV.13 General anaesthesia for Caesarian section:
A predisposes to low gastric pH
B should not include the use of volatile anaesthetic agents
C is contra-indicated in patients with a bleeding diathesis
D is a major cause of maternal mortality in labour
E should not include the use of atracurium.

IV.14 Placental blood flow is:
A independent of mean arterial blood pressure
B dependent upon local autoregulation
C reduced in hypoxia
D reduced by enflurane
E increased by isoflurane.

IV.15 Appropriate techniques in the treatment of eclampsia include:
A thiopentone infusion
B lumbar epidural anaesthesia
C trimethaphan infusion
D intravenous clonazepam
E emergency Caesarian section.

IV.16 Suitable intravenous doses of drugs for use during anaesthesia in a 3-year-old child include:
A neostigmine 0.08 mg/kg
B atropine 0.02 mg/kg
C d-tubocurarine 0.15 mg/kg
D alcuronium 0.6 mg/kg
E pethidine 0.25 mg/kg.

IV.17 Mydriasis during anaesthesia is produced by:

A pentolinium
B atropine
C naloxone
D promethazine
E dopamine.

IV.18 Non-depolarizing neuromuscular blocking drugs may be:

A potentiated by edrophonium
B ineffective in renal failure
C contra-indicated in myasthenia gravis
D reversed by physostigmine
E potentiated by aminoglycoside antibiotics.

IV.19 Interactions with drugs commonly used during anaesthesia should be expected with:

A imipramine
B chlordiazepoxide
C phenelzine
D neomycin
E levodopa.

IV.20 Low levels of serum cholinesterase are associated with:

A hepatic disease
B albuminuria
C the third trimester of pregnancy
D cardiac failure
E procaine therapy.

IV.21 Factors likely to contribute to the development of post-operative hepatic failure include:

A hypertension
B hypoxia
C blood transfusion
D hypercapnoea
E septicaemia.

IV.22 During one lung anaesthesia:

A inspired oxygen concentrations should be increased to at least 70%
B hyperoxic shunting reduces arterial pO_2
C CO_2 production is increased
D airway pressure increases
E halothane is contra-indicated.

IV.23 After left lower lobectomy:

- **A** apical and basal chest drains are both allowed to bubble under water
- **B** mediastinal flap occurs
- **C** the left heart border can no longer be delineated on the chest radiograph
- **D** atrial fibrillation may occur
- **E** thoracic epidural anaesthesia is contra-indicated.

IV.24 Block of the ulnar nerve at the elbow:

- **A** has a high incidence of neuritis
- **B** gives anaesthesia of the ulnar aspect of forearm and hand
- **C** will miss the posterior division
- **D** will not affect grip
- **E** will not reliably give anaesthesia of the ring finger (4th digit).

IV.25 The following are true of the blood supply in the arm:

- **A** the radial artery is usually larger than the ulnar artery
- **B** the radial artery is usually palpated lateral to the tendon of flexor carpi ulnaris
- **C** the radial artery helps form the deep palmar arch
- **D** the ulnar artery crosses the flexor retinaculum
- **E** the ulnar nerve lies medial to the ulnar artery at the wrist.

IV.26 The following are true of the 'typical' vertebra:

- **A** the pattern is that of a mid-thoracic vertebra
- **B** the spinal canal is bounded laterally by the pedicles and posteriorly by the laminae
- **C** the rib tubercles articulate with the transverse processes
- **D** the rib heads articulate with the vertebral bodies
- **E** the segmental nerve emerge below the corresponding vertebra.

IV.27 Concerning the arteries at the base of the brain:

- **A** the internal carotid becomes the middle cerebral
- **B** the anterior communicating is the anterior anastomotic connection between the internal carotid systems
- **C** the posterior communicating arteries join the internal carotids to the basilar
- **D** the posterior communicating arteries are absent in 12–18% of the population
- **E** the internal carotid lies lateral to the optic nerve.

IV.28 The inferior dental nerve:

- **A** is a sensory nerve
- **B** can be blocked as it enters the mandibular foramen above and behind the 3rd molar
- **C** when blocked, will give anaesthesia of all the ipsilateral lower teeth
- **D** successful block is likely to give partial anaesthesia of the tongue
- **E** ends by supplying sensation to the skin of the lower lip.

IV.29 Femoral nerve block:

- **A** is useful in reducing the pain of a fractured neck of femur
- **B** is part of the field block for repair of a femoral hernia
- **C** can be accomplished with 20 ml 2% lignocaine with adrenaline medial to the femoral artery just below the inguinal ligament
- **D** will allow operations on the patella
- **E** should not be performed in patients with arteriosclerotic disease of the leg

IV.30 Considering the brachial plexus:

- **A** it is primarily a plexus of sensory nerves
- **B** the cords are named from their relation to the axillary artery
- **C** there may be contributions from C4 and T2
- **D** anomalous cervical supply is often associated with anomalies of the first rib
- **E** block at the level of the first rib is more likely than the axillary approach to give good anaesthesia of the posterior cord (radial distribution).

IV.31 A blood urea concentration of 13 mmol/l occurs in:

- **A** dehydration
- **B** gastro-intestinal haemorrhage
- **C** pyloric stenosis
- **D** congestive cardiac failure
- **E** water intoxication

IV.32 The following occur in water retention:

- **A** an increase in the central venous pressure
- **B** inappropriate concentration of urine
- **C** an increase in body weight
- **D** hypernatraemia
- **E** a plasma osmolarity of 310 mmol/l.

IV.33 Secondary causes of cardiomyopathy include:

- **A** thyrotoxicosis
- **B** porphyria
- **C** dystrophia myotonica
- **D** alcoholism
- **E** prolonged artificial ventilation.

IV.34 Causes of sinus tachycardia include:

- **A** thyrotoxicosis
- **B** constrictive pericarditis
- **C** anaemia
- **D** nodal rhythm
- **E** mitral stenosis

IV.35 In a patient with severe arteriosclerosis:

- **A** autoregulation of renal blood flow is seriously impaired
- **B** if atropine is given as premedication, there is no particular need to reduce the dose
- **C** droperidol is contra-indicated
- **D** pre-operative treatment with beta-adrenergic blocking drugs should be discontinued at least 24 hours pre-operatively
- **E** induced hypotension is contra-indicated.

IV.36 A 40-year-old woman complains of increasing dyspnoea over 5 years. At cardiac catheterization she is found to have a systemic arterial pressure of 110/70, a pulmonary artery pressure of 80/40, a right atrial pressure of 5, a pulmonary capillary wedge pressure of 9, a right ventricular pressure of 80/5 and a left ventricular pressure of 110/8. These results are compatible with a diagnosis/ses of:

- **A** mitral stenosis
- **B** constrictive pericarditis
- **C** mitral insufficiency
- **D** primary myocardial disease
- **E** idiopathic pulmonary hypertension.

IV.37 In partial right-bundle branch block:

- **A** the QRS complex is wider than normal
- **B** S-waves are slurred in leads I, V5 and V6
- **C** there is ST depression in chest leads V1 and V2
- **D** there is T-wave inversion in leads V1 and V2
- **E** P-waves are inverted.

IV.38 A 40-year-old woman is to undergo routine cholecystectomy. She takes sulphasalazine and 3 mg of prednisolone per day for ulcerative colitis. The following are true:

A there is an aetiological connection between ulcerative colitis and gallstones
B there is an aetiological connection between steroid therapy and gallstones
C she should be given hydrocortisone with her premedication
D she should be given hydrocortisone 6 hours post-operatively
E additional potassium should be added to her post-operative intravenous fluids.

IV.39 Symptoms of a thyroid crisis include:

A fever
B bronchospasm
C abdominal pain
D cardiac arrhythmias
E coma.

IV.40 Generalized lymphadenopathy occurs in:

A rubella
B tuberculosis
C Still's disease
D disseminated lupus erythematosus
E sarcoidosis.

IV.41 Complications of diverticular disease likely to require surgical intervention include:

A haemorrhage
B vesicovaginal fistula
C stricture formation
D small-bowel obstruction
E anaemia

IV.42 Persistent vomiting is associated with:

A pancreatitis
B intussusception
C uraemia
D raised intracranial pressure
E hiatus hernia.

IV.43 In a patient with chronic hepatic disease:

A the action of suxamethonium is prolonged
B excretion of opiates is delayed
C vitamin K absorption is reduced
D prothrombin time is prolonged
E requirements for non-depolarizing neuromuscular blocking drugs are reduced.

IV.44 Causes of iron deficiency anaemia include::

A rheumatoid arthritis
B haemorrhage
C uraemia
D malabsorption
E thalassaemia.

IV.45 Eaton-Lambert syndrome:

A is a complication of bronchogenic carcinoma
B affects similar muscle groups to those involved in myasthenia gravis
C is associated with diminished tendon reflexes
D is reversed by intravenous anticholinesterases
E is not improved by surgery.

IV.46 The cardinal symptoms and signs of raised intracranial pressure include:

A loss of peripheral vision
B projectile vomiting
C bradycardia
D vertigo with vertical nystagmus
E a change of mental state.

IV.47 Drugs that can cause jaundice include:

A methyldopa
B tetracycline
C quinine
D diazepam
E penicillin.

IV.48 In renal ischaemia:

A urine volume is increased
B urinary sodium is decreased
C urinary creatinine is decreased
D urine output becomes directly proportional to blood pressure
E dobutamine selectively improves urine output.

IV.49 The following are features of chronic renal failure:

A bleeding tendency
B macrocytic anaemia
C hypertension
D splenomegaly
E tetany

IV.50 Hyperventilation leading to a lowered pCO_2 causes:

A a reduced cardiac output
B vasodilation of the cerebral blood vessels
C increased muscular excitability
D analgesia
E unconsciousness.

IV.51 Common causes of haemoptysis include:

A Goodpasture's syndrome
B bronchiectasis
C mitral stenosis
D pulmonary infarction
E Mallory-Weiss syndrome.

IV.52 The following signs would be likely in a patient with an acute exacerbation of chronic bronchitis:

A muscle twitching
B papilloedema
C bounding pulse
D reduced pulse pressure
E cold peripheries.

IV.53 A 60-year-old man complains of acute abdominal pain following a proven anterolateral myocardial infarction. The systolic blood pressure is 80 mm Hg, bowel sounds are absent and the abdomen is distended. Likely diagnoses include:

A acute cholecystitis
B superior mesenteric artery embolism
C diverticulitis of sigmoid colon
D acute pancreatitis
E perforated peptic ulcer.

IV.54 Surgical methods commonly used in the emergency treatment of bleeding oesophageal varices include:

A oesophageal transection
B sclerotherapy
C intravenous vasopressin therapy
D portacaval shunt
E splenectomy.

IV.55 Following splenectomy:

A there is an initial leucocytosis
B an initial phase of hypocoagulability is followed by hypercoagulability
C in infants there is an increased risk of pneumococcal pneumonia
D there is an increased incidence of portal hypertension
E tolerance to severe exercise is reduced because of reduced oxygen availability.

IV.56 Clinical features of small-bowel obstruction include:

A constant central abdominal pain made worse on movement
B nausea and vomiting
C dullness to percussion in the flanks
D abdominal distension
E absent bowel sounds.

IV.57 In the differential diagnosis between diverticulitis and carcinoma of the colon, the following would favour diverticulitis:

A weight loss
B abdominal pain
C episodes of profuse bleeding
D a palpable mass in the left iliac fossa
E a long history.

IV.58 The following are true of acute pancreatitis:

A the acute phase usually follows 2–3 weeks of prodromal symptoms
B fluid restriction is advisable in the early stages
C the patient may need repeated calcium supplements
D overall mortality is about 20%
E pancreatic pseudocyst is a rare complication.

IV.59 Dislocation of the shoulder:

A usually results in anterior displacement
B usually prevents the patient using the arm at all
C may cause paralysis of the deltoid
D requires general anaesthesia for reduction
E if recurrent, tends to occur on external rotation.

IV.60 After ureterocolic anastomosis:

A osteomalacia is a feature
B there is a hyperchloraemic acidosis
C patients should take extra salt
D there is hypokalaemia
E pyelonephritis is rare because of ureteric peristalsis.

Paper IV Answers

IV.1 **TTTTT**

IV.2 **TTTTT**

A–E None of these has been specifically implicated as a trigger of malignant hyperpyrexia and all are recommended for use in susceptible patients.

IV.3 **TTFFF**

A These patients are often too difficult for local anaesthesia.

B Local anaesthesia does not work well in the presence of infection.

C,D,E All are relative contra-indications to general anaesthesia, whether in the dental chair or not.

IV.4 **TFTFT**

B Suxamethonium is contra-indicated if there is potential obstruction of the airway.

D Blind nasal intubation during spontaneous ventilation is probably the technique of choice.

IV.5 **FTFFF**

A This will only kill bacteria, not spores.

C Ethylene oxide will kill spores too if left for long enough.

D It needs 10–12 hours.

E Chlorhexidine takes 20, not 3, minutes!

IV.6 **TTTFT**

D Acidosis; all precipitating factors are related to impaired cellular oxygenation.

IV.7 **TTTFT**

D Bradycardia usually, due to vagal stimulation.

IV.8 **TTTFF**

D Unconnected.

E There is said to be a reduced incidence of pulmonary problems after spinal as opposed to general anaesthesia.

IV.9 **FFTFT**

A,B Insufficient content of factor VIII.

D This is an antifibrinolytic and not suitable for treatment of haemophilia.

IV.10 **FFTTF**

A Not used.

D Used to cause peripheral vasodilation — with care that the circulating blood volume is maintained.

B,E Not a treatment for septicaemia, although it may be considered if DIC develops.

IV.11 TTFFF

C Not immediate routine therapy is casualty.
B Certainly not as first-line treatment.
E Resuscitate first, and then the attack, if it is the cause, will recover.

IV.12 TFTTT

B Produce meiosis.
E Due to pupillary and respiratory effects.

IV.13 FFFTF

A General anaesthesia does not reduce the pH of gastric contents.
B Low-dose halothane or enflurane is satisfactory.
C The diathesis should be treated if possible; epidural anaesthesia would be contra-indicated.
D General anesthesia, per se, is an important, and often preventable, cause of death.
E Atracurium is probably the best non-depolarizer to use; there is certainly no reason to avoid it unless an idiosyncrasy is suspected in the patient.

IV.14 FFTTF

A Is reduced in hypotension.
B No local autoregulatory mechanisms.
E Uterine vessels are normally dilated, and so a vasodilator would have little effect.

IV.15 TTTTT

A,D For fitting.
B,C To reduce the blood pressure.
E The only known cure for pre-eclampsia and eclampsia is delivery.

IV.16 TTFFT

C 0.5 mg/ kg d-tubocurarine.
D Up to 0.3 mg/kg alcuronium.

IV.17 TFFFF

B Systemic atropine has no effect at normal dosage.
C Only prevents opiate-induced meiosis.
D,E No effect.

IV.18 FFTTT

A Antagonized: edrophonium is an anti-cholinesterase.
B If affected at all by renal function, blockers will be potentiated because of reduced excretion.

IV.19 FFTTT

A Tricyclic antidepressant, which may produce enzyme induction but will not cause adverse interactions.
B Benzodiazepine
C MAOI.
D Interference with neuromuscular blockade.
E Converted to dopamine in the basal ganglia, there is a risk of dysrhythmias with halothane. There may also be interaction with droperidol, which is a central dopamine antagonist.

IV.20 TFTTF

B Serum cholinesterase levels are not reduced by albuminuria per se.
E They are not reduced, it is just that procaine will compete with suxamethonium for metabolism by plasma cholinesterase.

IV.21 FTTTT

A HYPOtension predisposes to impaired hepatic perfusion and oxygenation.

IV.22 FTFTF

A Not necessarily; it depends upon the individual patient's lung function.
C CO_2 production depends upon metabolism, not ventilation.
D Compliance will be reduced and airway pressure will increase unless tidal volume is reduced.
E Is indicated for its vasodilator properties in the pulmonary circulation.

IV.23 TFFTF

B Not, provided the remaining lung is expanded.
C Not if the left upper lobe is expanded.
E No, may provide good post-operative analgesia.

IV.24 TFFFT

There are no branches of the ulnar above the elbow (**C**); the medial aspect of the forearm is supplied by cutaneous branches from the medial cord (**B**).

D The ulnar nerve supplies many of the small muscles of the hand.
E There is individual variation.

IV.25 FTTTT

A The radial artery is the more direct continuation of the brachial and is the choice for cannulation, but the ulnar artery is usually the larger.
C It anastomoses with the deep branch of the ulnar artery.

IV.26 TTTTT

B With the spinous process this makes up the neural arch.
E The cervical nerves emerge above the vertebrae, but the question asks of the 'typical' vertebra.

IV.27 TTFFT

A Via the anterior cerebral arteries.
C They are the anastomotic connections between the areas of supply, but the arteries actually join the internal carotids to the posterior cerebrals.

IV.28 FTTTT

A Supplies muscles in the floor of the mouth before it enters the mandibular foramen.

D Because the lingual nerve is close by.

E As the mental nerve.

IV.29 TFFFF

A Note the question does not say 'abolish'.

B There is no femoral distribution this proximal.

C All correct except that the nerve is lateral to the artery.

D Will need obturator and, probably, lateral cutaneous nerve of thigh.

E Solutions containing vasoconstrictors should be used with care.

IV.30 FTTTT

A No!!! — there is no separation of motor and sensory.

IV.31 TTFTF

B Absorption and breakdown of haemoglobin increase the plasma urea.

C Produces a metabolic alkalosis, but not uraemia.

D A reasonably likely event because of reduced renal perfusion in a state of low cardiac output.

E Would be low if anything.

IV.32 FTTFF

A Not likely, unless there is also sodium retention.

D,E There will be hyponatraemia and reduced plasma osmolarity.

IV.33 TTTFF

D Alcohol causes a primary cardiomyopathy.
E Not described.

IV.34 TTTFF

D,E Not causes of sinus tachycardia: nodal rhythm must be generated by the A–V node; mitral stenosis can precipitate atrial fibrillation.

IV.35 TTFFT

C No, droperidol is if anything cardiovascularly stable.
D Therapy should be maintained up to the time of operation.
E Large falls in blood pressure may compromise the cerebral or coronary circulation.

IV.36 FFFFT

When stems give data, think about possible diagnoses before looking at the branches.

A,B,C,D Normal pressures are found in the right and left atria, the left ventricle and the aorta — the only abnormal findings are hypertension in the right ventricle and pulmonary artery.

IV.37 FTTTF

A The QRS complex is wide if RBBB is complete but, unlike in LBBB, is not always widened.
E Atrial conduction is unaffected.

IV.38 FFFFF

A,B There is no aetiological connection between ulcerative colitis or steroid therapy and gallstones.

C,D 3 mg of prednisolone is well below a suppressant dose.

E There is no special need for potassium.

IV.39 TFTTF

B Not a feature of thyroid crisis.

E Cerebral excitation, rather than coma.

IV.40 TTTTT

C Juvenile rheumatoid arthritis.

D In 45% of cases.

IV.41 TTTTF

E Although a common complication of diverticular disease, it would not itself indicate operation — haemorrhage, on the other hand, would do so.

IV.42 TTTTF

E Usually regurgitation or intermittent vomiting.

IV.43 FTFTT

A Only if there is gross failure of hepatic function.
C Not unless jaundice is present.

IV.44 FTFTF

A,C,E Although these may produce a hypochromic anaemia, it is not iron-deficient and is more commonly normochromic.

IV.45 TFTFF

B Peripheral muscular weakness rather than central.
D Not affected.
E May improve with resection of the primary tumour.

IV.46 FTTFT

The cardinal features are (**B,C,E**), papilloedema and morning headaches. That is not to say that someone with raised ICP cannot have loss of vision or vertigo, but these are localizing signs.

IV.47 TTTFT

D Not an established cause of jaundice.

IV.48 FTTFF

A Decreased — the question does not suggest polyuric failure.
D Depends upon oxygenation.
E Dopamine is the selective agent; dobutamine increases urine output by increasing cardiac output.

IV.49 TFTFF

B Microcytic anaemia, not macrocytic, with chronic renal failure.

E Tetany occurs in alkalosis and is associated with low ionized calcium. Chronic renal failure tends to acidosis and hypercalcaemia.

IV.50 TFTTT

B Cerebral vasoconstriction.

C Respiratory alkalosis leading to tetany.

IV.51 FTTTF

A Goodpasture's syndrome (when it occurs) commonly causes haemoptysis, but it is rare!

E This may mimic haemoptysis, but is due to persistent vomiting.

IV.52 TTTFF

Question I.52 was similar.

C,D A bounding pulse usually indicates a wide pulse pressure.

E Carbon dioxide retention is responsible for many of the signs, amongst which are warm peripheries caused by vasodilatation.

IV.53 FTFFT

The key words are: 'after a PROVEN myocardial infarction' and 'LIKELY diagnoses'.

A,C,D Not particularly likely, and do not adequately explain the distension and paralytic ileus (except, possibly, pancreatitis).

E Probably a reasonable alternative in a man of this age.

IV.54 TTFFF

C Not a surgical method.

D Although used to reduce portal hypertension, it is not routinely used to treat bleeding varices.

E Would not prevent bleeding and may elevate pressure further.

IV.55 TFTFT

- **B** There is an increased platelet count and hypercoagulability.
- **C** Infants should be given anti-pneumococcal vaccine prior to splenectomy.
- **D** No association.
- **E** The spleen does not hold a significant volume of blood reserve in humans, and the oxygen-combining characteristics are unchanged after splenectomy.

IV.56 FTFTF

- **A** Abdominal pain is usually colicky rather than constant.
- **C** Obstruction produces gaseous distension which is resonant — dullness in the flanks is due to fluid (ascites) or blood.
- **E** Bowel sounds are tinkling; sounds are absent in paralytic ileus.

IV.57 FTTFT

- **A** Weight loss makes a cancer more likely.
- **C** Bleeding from carcinoma is usually in small amounts.
- **D** A mass may be palpable in both conditions (which may anyway co-exist); a tender mass favours diverticulitis.

IV.58 FFTTF

- **A** There are not usually prodromal symptoms.
- **B** Fluid losses are large and must be replaced.
- **E** It is a common complication, thought it doesn't always need operative intervention.

IV.59 TTTFT

- **B** Pain usually prevents movement after a dislocation of the shoulder.
- **C** The circumflex nerve may be damaged.
- **D** Reduction is often possible with sedation and analgesia. Interscalene block of the brachial plexus is another technique.

IV.60 TTFTF

- **C** Patients should reduce their salt intake.
- **E** Pyelonephritis is almost inevitable. A conduit avoids these problems.

Paper V Questions

V.1 Agents which may safely be used during anaesthesia in a child who was badly burned 4 days previously include:

A thiopentone.
B halothane
C suxamethonium
D atracarium
E ketamine.

V.2 Untreated pre-operative hypertension:

A is associated with an increased incidence of peri-operative myocardial infarction
B should be treated before surgery
C is a contra-indication to the use of halothane
D predisposes to deep venous thrombosis
E precludes the intra-operative use of sodium nitroprusside.

V.3 In a poorly controlled diabetic on glibenclamide therapy presenting for amputation of an infected great toe:

A surgery should be postponed if the patient is ketotic
B pre-operative therapy should include an infusion containing dextrose and insulin
C serum potassium is likely to be elevated
D halothane should be avoided
E spinal anaesthesia is contra-indicated.

V.4 In a 5-year-old child undergoing general anaesthesia for elective adenotonsillectomy:

A nasal intubation is preferable to allow optimal surgical access
B a Boyle-Davis gag is contra-indicated
C thiopentone should not be used because of the risk of apnoea
D throat packs are frequently not used
E premedication should be with atropine alone to minimize post-operative sedation.

V.5 Regarding endotracheal intubation:

A endotracheal insufflation was first described in the 17th century
B John Snow first described intubation of a tracheostomy in 1858
C blind nasal intubation was pioneered by Magill and Rowbotham in the 1940s
D the Magill laryngoscope blade is designed to lift the epiglottis forward
E the Rowbotham angle-piece was specifically designed for insertion of a suction catheter.

V.6 Factors which increase the likelihood of regurgitation at induction include:

A obesity
B anxiety
C upper respiratory obstruction
D raised 'barrier' pressure
E atropine premedication.

V.7 With regard to the basic principles of anaesthesia

A the triad of anaesthesia was first described in 1900
B the three basic components of anaesthesia are narcosis, reflex suppression and analgesia
C the two agents which satisfactorily provide all three parts of the triad are ether and cyclopropane
D halothane has no analgesic properties
E balanced anaesthesia was first described by Lundy in 1926.

V.8 Likely causes of post-operative jaundice include:

A blood transfusion
B halothane hepatitis
C sphincteric spasm
D post-operative pancreatitis
E renal failure

V.9 In a patient suffering from sickle-cell trait:

A 30–40% of the total haemoglobin is haemoglobin S
B sickling occurs with a PaO_2 less than 45 mm Hg
C the use of tourniquets is contra-indicated
D pre-operative transfusion is indicated if the haemoglobin concentration is less than 10 g per 100 ml
E acidosis is harmful because of the resulting right shift of the oxyhaemoglobin dissociation curve.

V.10 A 23-year-old motorcyclist is brought into casualty unconscious. His blood pressure is 80/40 and his pulse rate is 115. He has no broken limbs and clinically he has fractured lower right ribs.
The following are true:

- **A** the most likely cause of the cardiovascular signs is a tension pneumothorax
- **B** cyanosis may be caused by adult respiratory distress syndrome
- **C** he could be unconscious because of hypotension
- **D** the fast pulse indicates that the intracranial pressure is not raised
- **E** urgent laparotomy is indicated.

V.11 Late complications of orotracheal intubation include:

- **A** granuloma pyogenicum
- **B** tracheal stenosis
- **C** recurrent laryngeal nerve injury
- **D** bronchopleural fistula
- **E** dysphonia.

V.12 The following would be suitable doses in a fit 80 kg man:

- **A** 25 ml 1.5% lignocaine + adrenaline caudally for haemorrhoidectomy
- **B** 40 ml 0.5% plain bupivacaine epidurally for bilateral herniorraphy
- **C** 2.5 ml 0.5% hyperbaric cinchocaine intrathecally for transurethral resection of prostate
- **D** 0.6 ml 0.5% hyperbaric cinchocaine intrathecally with patient sitting for anal stretch
- **E** 40 ml 1.5% lignocaine with adrenaline epidurally at L2–3 for cholecystectomy.

V.13 Cerebral blood flow:

- **A** is directly related to cardiac output
- **B** is posturally dependent
- **C** is reduced when bleeding drops pressure down to 80 mm Hg systolic
- **D** is autoregulated between mean pressures of 40 and 180 mm Hg
- **E** represents 30% of the cardiac output.

V.14 During the last trimester of pregnancy:

- **A** lung compliance is decreased
- **B** haematocrit is increased
- **C** blood volume is increased
- **D** gastric secretion is increased
- **E** total peripheral resistance is reduced.

V.15 Concerning the nerve supply to the pregnant uterus:

A sensation from the upper segment travels with the sympathetic nerves to T11 and T12

B sensation from the birth canal is transmitted via the pudendal nerve

C sensation from the lower segment travels via L2,3,4

D motor function is served by both sympathetic and parasympathetic nerves

E an intact nerve supply is essential to initiate the process of normal labour.

V.16 Symptoms or signs likely to occur in amniotic fluid embolism include:

A cyanosis

B hypofibrinogenaemia

C chest pain

D hypoventilation

E hypertension.

V.17 Likely causes of postoperative apnoea in a neonate include:

A hypothermia

B inadequate reversal of neuromuscular blockade

C concurrent intravenous antibiotic therapy

D hypotension

E hypoglycaemia.

V.18 The following statements are true:

A the action of hyoscine is longer than atropine

B both atropine and hyoscine increase pulmonary dead space

C atropine premedication is contra-indicated in febrile children

D 4.0 mg atropine is required to produce complete vagal blockade in a 70 kg man

E hyoscine premedication is contra-indicated in elderly patients.

V.19 The ventilatory depressant effects of morphine can be countered by:

A inhalation of 5% carbon dioxide in oxygen

B infusion of physostigmine

C intravenous levorphanol

D intravenous naloxone

E infusion of doxapram.

V.20 Atropine is used in premedication:

A to antagonize parasympathetic activity
B for its anti-emetic effect
C for its sedative action
D because it increases hepatic clearance of anaesthetic agents
E to prevent surgically induced dysrhythmias.

V.21 High levels of serum cholinesterase occur with:

A alcoholism
B ecothiopate therapy
C pregnancy
D thyrotoxicosis
E obesity.

V.22 Concerning the flammability of anaesthetic gases

A halothane is non-flammable at atmospheric pressure
B the minimal flammable concentration of diethyl ether in oxygen is 2.1%
C spontaneous ignition can occur if oxygen under pressure comes into contact with grease
D the minimum temperature which will ignite a potentially explosive anaesthetic mixture is 96°C
E the halothane–ether azeotrope is non-flammable in oxygen up to a concentration of 7.5%.

V.23 During one-lung anaesthesia, the use of halothane:

A increases carbon dioxide production
B increases ventilation/perfusion mismatching
C increases pulmonary vascular resistance
D may precipitate cardiac arrhythmias
E increases airway pressure.

V.24 The following are true of the nose and nasal cavity:

A the medial wall of the nasal cavity is partly cartilaginous
B there are three separate turbinate bones
C the best route for nasal intubation is below the inferior turbinate
D the paranasal sinuses are not fully developed until adolescence
E septoplasty can be performed under topical analgesia.

V.25 The following are true of the nerve supply to the arm:

- **A** the musculocutaneous (C5,6) supplies skin between mid-upper arm and the lateral epicondyle
- **B** the lateral cutaneous nerve of forearm (C5,6) suplies skin between the lateral epicondyle and the base of the thumb
- **C** the hand should be kept pronated if the arm is abducted in an anaesthetized subject
- **D** the median nerve passes beneath the flexor retinaculum at the wrist
- **E** the circumflex nerve is susceptible to injury as it traverses the spiral groove of the humerus.

V.26 The femoral artery:

- **A** is the continuation of the external iliac
- **B** is readily palpable throughout its length
- **C** is separated from the hip joint only by the tendon of psoas major
- **D** lies medial to the femoral nerve just below the inguinal ligament
- **E** in some subjects follows an aberrant course and is known as the profunda femoris.

V.27 The following are true of the sacrum:

- **A** it consists of five fused vertebrae
- **B** the sacral hiatus represents the absent last neural arch
- **C** the hiatus is the caudal limit of the extradural space
- **D** the anatomy is constant between individuals
- **E** the capacity of the adult sacral canal is 20–25 ml.

V.28 The following are true of the oculomotor nerve:

- **A** it runs through the cavernous sinus into the superior orbital fissure
- **B** it supplies sympathetic and parasympathetic innervation to the eye
- **C** fibres subserving reflex activity synapse in the superior colliculus
- **D** a palsy results in a 'relaxed' pupil, fixed at mid-dilatation
- **E** a palsy results in a convergent squint.

V.29 Damage to the facial nerve during a superficial parotidectomy:

- **A** can be prevented by avoiding the use of non-depolarizing muscle relaxants
- **B** will result in partial loss of corneal sensation
- **C** will result in partial facial paralysis
- **D** will result in loss of sweating over the affected part
- **E** will result in partial loss of taste.

V.30 The medial popliteal (tibial) nerve:

A is the larger of the two terminal branches of the sciatic nerve
B supplies the muscles of the calf
C gives an articular division to the knee
D subserves sensation over the posterolateral aspect of lower leg and foot via the sural nerve
E terminates by dividing into the medial and lateral plantar nerves that supply sensation to the sole of the foot.

V.31 The cervical plexus:

A is formed by the anterior primary rami after each has emerged lateral to the vertebral artery
B receives a branch (the ansa hypoglossi) from the 12th cranial nerve
C supplies cutaneous sensation to the anterior chest wall down to the third rib.
D supplies motor fibres to levator scapulae, sternomastoid and trapezius
E supplies sensation to the forehead via the anterior auricular branch of the lesser occipital nerve.

V.32 Clinical findings consistent with persistent vomiting for two months include:

A vitamin B_{12} deficiency anaemia
B a blood urea of 12 mmol/l
C hypokalaemia
D hypochloraemia
E tetany.

V.33 In coarctation of the aorta:

A notching is best seen in the first and second ribs
B girls are more commonly affected than boys
C intra-operative hypotension is best treated with halothane
D there is an association with a bicuspid aortic valve
E it is best to treat conservatively until after 20 years of age.

V.34 Causes of syncope include:

A diabetes
B aortic incompetence
C hypertrophic obstructive cardiomyopathy
D coughing
E hypercapnoea.

V.35 A slow regular pulse is associated with:
- **A** complete heart block
- **B** idioventricular rhythm
- **C** nodal rhythm
- **D** a 2:1 atrioventricular block
- **E** constrictive pericarditis.

V.36 Suitable treatment for paroxysmal atrial tachycardia includes:
- **A** beta-adrenergic blockade
- **B** anticholinesterase therapy
- **C** carotid sinus massage
- **D** vasopressin
- **E** intravenous lignocaine.

V.37 When atrial fibrillation complicates mitral stenosis:
- **A** there are prominent 'a' waves in the jugular venous pulse
- **B** closed mitral valvotomy is contra-indicated
- **C** long-term anticoagulation is indicated
- **D** left ventricular failure frequently occurs
- **E** a systolic murmur is not present.

V.38 In the Wolff-Parkinson-White syndrome:
- **A** there is a short PR interval on the ECG
- **B** heart failure never occurs
- **C** beta-adrenergic blockers are indicated
- **D** the patient can terminate the attacks by manoeuvres that increase vagal tone
- **E** a cardiac pacemaker may be needed.

V.39 The following are true of hypoglycaemic coma:
- **A** the patient is likely to be sweaty
- **B** the pupils are dilated
- **C** the pulse volume is good
- **D** it is a feature of Addison's disease
- **E** glucagon can be given intramuscularly.

V.40 Concerning acromegaly:
- **A** there is proximal muscle weakness
- **B** it is a cause of hepatosplenomegaly
- **C** Paget's disease deforms the skull
- **D** bromocriptine is used in treatment
- **E** despite intubation problems, anaesthesia is well tolerated.

V.41 Splenomegaly occurs in:

- A tuberculosis
- B hereditary spherocytosis
- C porphyria
- D carcinoma of the head of the pancreas
- E thyrotoxicosis

V.42 Ulcerative colitis:

- A predisposes the sufferer to the development of sarcomas of the large bowel
- B medical treatment includes immunosuppression and steroids
- C colectomy should include excision of the rectum
- D is associated with hepatic dysfunction
- E is usually a self-limiting condition.

V.43 Causes of diffuse hepatomegaly include:

- A haemochromatosis
- B tricuspid incompetence
- C constrictive pericarditis
- D myelofibrosis
- E tuberculosis.

V.44 A haemoglobin of 8 g/100 ml with a reticulocyte count of 10% occurs in:

- A aplastic anaemia
- B untreated pernicious anaemia
- C polycythaemia
- D haemolytic anaemia
- E acute leukaemia.

V.45 In a patient with known myasthenia gravis and progressive weakness:

- A intravenous neostigmine will produce immediate improvement
- B hypokalaemia may be a contributing factor
- C all oral medication should be temporarily withdrawn
- D thymectomy is indicated
- E atropine will produce symptomatic improvement.

V.46 Polyneuropathy is a recognized feature of:

- A myaesthenia gravis
- B mercury poisoning
- C alcoholism
- D polyarteritis nodosa
- E bronchogenic carcinoma.

V.47 Methaemoglobinaemia occurs secondary to treatment with:

- **A** sulphonamides
- **B** procaine
- **C** sodium nitroprusside
- **D** phenacetin
- **E** sodium nitrite.

V.48 Peri-operative oliguria is related to:

- **A** antidiuretic hormone release
- **B** stimulation of aldosterone release
- **C** the third space effect
- **D** a specific effect of anaesthesia on renal tubules
- **E** hyperglycaemia.

V.49 Features of acute glomerulonephritis include:

- **A** oliguria
- **B** hypertension
- **C** peri-orbital oedema
- **D** early onset of ascites
- **E** haematuria.

V.50 A reduction in the diffusing capacity of the lung occurs in:

- **A** emphysema
- **B** polycythaemia
- **C** pulmonary embolism
- **D** anaemia
- **E** anaesthesia for elective cholecystectomy.

V.51 The development of a spontaneous pneumothorax is associated with;

- **A** congenital lung bullae
- **B** cigarette smoking
- **C** rheumatoid arthritis
- **D** hydatid lung disease
- **E** asthma.

V.52 Blood for gas analysis is taken from a patient with an acute exacerbation of chronic bronchitis. Which of these results are compatible with this diagnosis?

- **A** PaO_2 5.6 kPa
- **B** $PaCO_2$ 10.4 kPa
- **C** pH 7.58
- **D** BE 8.3 mmol/l
- **E** S.Bic. 18 mmol/l.

V.53 A 49-year-old man arrives in casualty complaining of epigastric pain that radiates through to the back. He is dyspnoeic, centrally cyanosed, and has absent bowel sounds. Which are are likely diagnoses?

A acute pancreatitis
B dissecting aortic aneurysm
C myocardial infarction
D perforated duodenal ulcer
E ascending cholangitis.

V.54 Patients with advanced breast carcinoma likely to respond to hormone manipulation include those:

A over five years postmenopausal at the time of initial presentation
B with primarily soft tissue metastases
C with advanced local disease, but without metastases
D with a short recurrence-free interval
E with oestrogen receptor-positive tumours.

V.55 Indications for a portacaval shunt in portal hypertension include:

A repeated episodes of bleeding from varices
B increasing jaundice
C a falling serum albumin
D as prophylaxis to prevent bleeding in young patients
E recurring troublesome ascites.

V.56 Shortly after perforation of a duodenal ulcer:

A the axillary temperature is subnormal
B maximum tenderness is situated in the right iliac fossa
C shoulder pain occurs
D serum amylase is raised
E haemodilution occurs.

V.57 The following are features of acute appendicitis:

A pain is initially poorly localized
B persistent vomiting
C early development of pyrexia
D a leucocytosis of 10 000 cells per mm^3
E perforation is more likely in patients under 2 years old.

V.58 Features of chronic pyloric obstruction include:

A tetany
B visible peristalsis
C postural hypotension
D hypokalaemia
E epigastric succussion splash.

V.59 The following are true of a supracondylar fracture of the humerus:

A it is an injury that tends to occur in children
B nerve damage is uncommon
C closed reduction is usually satisfactory
D loss of the radial pulse is an indication for urgent surgery
E Volkmann's ischaemic contracture is a complication.

V.60 In benign prostatic hypertrophy:

A patients have to strain to start their stream
B frequency is the earliest symptom
C chronic retention should not be decompressed rapidly
D an excretory pyelogram should be obtained if there is renal failure
E an episode of acute retention is an indication for prostatectomy.

Paper V Answers

V.1 **TTFTT**

C Suxamethonium may cause hyperkalaemia after severe burns. The timespan quoted is usually the order of weeks after the burn, but the question says 'safely used'.

V.2 **FTFFF**

A Only if there is a recent history of myocardial infarction.
C Halothane helps stabilize blood pressure.
D No relationship.
E Nitroprusside may be required.

V.3 **FTFFF**

A Control will only be achieved after operative treatment.
C No reason why!
D,E Neither is contra-indicated.

V.4 **FFFTF**

A Nasal intubation is not normally used in young children, particularly if adenoidectomy is also to be performed.
B Commonly used, though in a modified form (Doughty blade).
C Not a contra-indication in an elective case.
E Sedative and analgesic premedication is preferable.

V.5 **TTFTF**

C During the 1920s.

E The Rowbotham angle-piece does not have a suction port.

V.6 **TTTFT**

D Regurgitation is LESS likely if the barrier pressure of the lower oesophageal sphincter is raised.

E Atropine reduces the tone of sphincters and the motility of the gut. However, in normal doses this is more a theoretical than a practical problem.

V.7 **FFFTT**

A 1950 by Rees and Gray.

B Reflex suppression and analgesia are similar; the third component is relaxation.

C Chloroform, not cyclopropane.

V.8 **TFTTF**

B Although this may occur, it is not a likely cause.

E May be associated, but is not a cause — careful!

V.9 **TTTFT**

D Not unless the patient is far more severely anaemic than this.

V.10 FFFFF

All these answers have a grain of truth in them, but they are all false.

A Bleeding: into abdomen or thorax, or from the head.
B Too early: more likely tension pneumothorax, aspiration or central respiratory depression because of head injury.
C A systolic pressure of 80 in a previously fit young man will not cause unconsciousness.
D Certainly not!
E There is need for laparotomy only if abdominal trauma is suspected (see comment **A**).

V.11 TTTFT

D Bronchopleural fistula is not a documented complication of orotracheal intubation.

V.12 TTFTT

There is no absolute 'correct dose'; the volume necessary will vary from patient to patient. Having said that:

B this is a large dose of bupivacaine, and would also need some head-down tilt;
C a TURP rarely needs more than 1.6 ml heavy cinchocaine;
E you may not choose this technique, but it is a suitable dose.

V.13 FFTFF

A Not directly related.
D Autoregulation applies between mean pressures of 60 and 140 mm Hg.
E 15% of cardiac output.

V.14 FFTFT

A Lung compliance increases.
B Haematocrit decreases and flow improves.
D Not increased, although gastric emptying is delayed.

V.15 TTFTF

C Via the sacral parasympathetics: S2–4.
E Normal labour can occur in patients with spinal cord transection.

V.16 TTTFF

D Acute hypoxia causes hyperventilation.
E Hypotension caused by cardiovascular collapse (peripheral vasodilation and myocardial depression).

V.17 TFTFT

The important word here is 'likely'.

B It may produce respiratory problems, but not apnoea.
D Hypotension would have to be very severe and therefore is not a likely cause.

V.18 TTTFT

B Bronchodilation increases bronchiolar volume and hence anatomical dead space.
D 2.0 mg atropine.
E Hyoscine can cause confusion in the elderly.

V.19 TFFTT

The question says 'countered', not 'reversed'.

A Perhaps not universally good clinical practice, but we do use CO_2 if patients are slow to breathe post-operatively — admittedly they may then be hypocarbic.
B Anticholinesterase.
C Levallorphan yes, but not levorphanol.

V.20 TFFFT

B Atropine, unlike hyoscine, is not an anti-emetic.
C Central stimulant.
D No evidence, and it is not an enzyme inducer.

V.21 TFFTT

B This is a cholinesterase inhibitor, so although it may only reduce the effect of serum cholinesterase, rather than the actual amount, it is certainly not associated with high levels of the enzyme.
C Low levels occur, particularly in the second half of pregnancy.

V.22 TTTFT

D 18°C.
E This is rarely used now: if you knew, then you pick up a bonus mark; don't worry if you didn't.

V.23 FFFTF

A If anything it will reduce CO_2 production by reducing metabolic rate.
B Either reduced or unchanged, due to vasodilation.
C Reduces it due to vasodilation.
E As a bronchodilator will lower it or have no effect.

V.24 TFTTF

B Only the inferior turbinate is separate: the upper and middle are part of the ethmoid.
E The base of the septum and the columella need the injection of some local anaesthetic because they are not covered by mucous membrane but by squamous epithelium.

V.25 FTTTF

A,B The musculocutaneous nerve terminates as the lateral cutaneous nerve of forearm.

C To help avoid damage to the brachial plexus.

E This is the radial nerve; the circumflex is susceptible to damage as it runs round the surgical neck of the humerus.

V.26 TFTTF

C An important point of applied anatomy: it is easy, especially in infants, to puncture the hip joint when attempting a femoral stab.

E The profunda femoris is a large vessel that is the main blood supply to the adductors, flexors and extensors of the thigh.

V.27 TTTFT

C The hiatus is roofed by the posterior sacro-coccygeal ligaments.

D The anatomy is notoriously variable, and that is a great nuisance to the anaesthetist.

V.28 TFTFF

B,D The oculomotor supplies PNS fibres. A palsy gives a dilated pupil because of unopposed SNS action.

E Divergent squint; the muscles NOT supplied are the lateral rectus and superior oblique.

V.29 FFTFF

A The use of relaxant has no influence of itself, but no relaxant (or allowing the relaxant to partially reverse) will enable the surgeon to use a nerve stimulator to identify the branches.

B,D Trigeminal.

E Too far distal to affect taste.

V.30 TTTTT

D Variable contribution from the lateral popliteal.
E The lateral plantar (equivalent of the ulnar in the hand) supplies most of the small muscles of the foot.

V.31 FFTTF

A C1 lies medial to the artery.
B The hypoglossal (XII) FORMS the ansa hypoglossi WITH contributions from C1–3.
D Sternomastoid and trapezius are mainly supplied from the spinal accessory (XI).
E The face is supplied by the trigeminal (V).

V.32 FTTTT

A Two months is not long enough in which to develop B_{12} deficiency.
B Dehydration.
C,D,E Metabolic alkalosis.

V.33 FFFTF

A It is the lower ribs which are contacted by the internal mammary artery.
B Predominantly males.
C Acute treatment requires direct acting vasodilators, e.g. sodium nitroprusside.
E Best treated earlier before hypertension has developed, but diagnosis is often delayed.

V.34 TFTTF

A Due to associated autonomic neuropathy.
B Aortic stenosis, not incompetence.
E Syncope occurs when hypocapnoea is caused by hysterical hyperventilation.

V.35 TTTTF

E Usually a sinus tachycardia, certainly not a slow pulse.

V.36 TFTFF

B Anticholinesterases are never used to cause bradycardia.

D Vasopressin is a synthetic ADH. It is used in diabetes insipidus and, in higher dosage, for its vasoconstricting properties in patients with bleeding varices. How could it help in a paroxysmal atrial tachycardia? A connection is that patients may have a diuresis following a paroxysm, but vasopressin is not used.

E Not good for supraventricular dysrhythmias.

V.37 FTFFT

A 'a' waves are absent in atrial fibrillation.

B Because of the risk of embolization.

C Not necessarily, although it used to be advocated more commonly.

D It could well supervene eventually, but the onset of AF is not a frequent cause.

E A catch: the implication is that, if AF is not present then there is a systolic murmur, but the murmur of mitral stenosis is a diastolic one!

V.38 TFTTT

B Almost nothing is 'never' or 'always' in medicine. Failure of output can occur in tachycardia.

E Pacemakers can be used in tachy-dysrhythmias but are not always as effective as they are in brady-arrhythmias.

V.39 TTTTT

A,B,C Signs of sympathetic overactivity.

E True, although intravenous glucose is the more usual approach.

V.40 TTFTF

C Overgrowth of bone occurs in acromegaly. Paget's disease has a different pathology.

E Acromegalics tolerate anaesthesia poorly.

V.41 **TTTTF**

D By occlusion of the portal vein.
E Thyrotoxicosis does not cause splenomegaly.

V.42 **FTTTF**

A Adenocarcinoma of the colon and rectum, hence **C**.
E It is usually a relapsing condition.

V.43 **TFTTT**

B Tricuspid stenosis and associated raised venous pressure.

V.44 **FFFTF**

A A reticulocyte count of 10% is too high for aplasia.
C Haemoglobin will be high in polycythaemia.
E Reticulocyte count will be low in acute leukaemia.

V.45 **FTTFF**

A Not necessarily; the patient may be in cholinergic crisis — remember, the question implies that the patient has already been diagnosed with the disease and so may be on treatment.
D Not as a first-line treatment for progressive weakness.
E Certainly not!

V.46 **FTTTT**

A A condition solely of the neuromuscular junction.
C Both because of the chronic alcohol intake and the associated malnutrition.
D A very rare condition.
E Lung cancer has many non-metastatic systemic manifestations and is a very common disease.

V.47 TFTTT

B Prilocaine, not procaine.

C Methaemoglobin is formed within the red cells as a result of SNP breakdown.

V.48 TFTFF

B Does not have a clinically measurable effect on peri-operative urine output.

D Not apart from direct nephrotoxicity.

E Hyperglycaemia, if anything, produces a diuresis.

V.49 TTTFT

B Hypertension is multi-factorial: increased extracellular fluid volume, increased cardiac output and an increased peripheral vascular resistance.

C,D Oedema may develop first peri-orbitally, but can eventually become generalized.

V.50 TFTTF

B Polycythaemia may be associated with increased diffusing capacity.

E Elective upper abdominal surgery does not alter diffusing capacity, though it may change FRC.

V.51 TFFTT

A Not a direct association; the association is via chronic bronchitis and emphysema.

C Not a feature of rheumatoid lung.

V.52 TTFTF

He will be acutely acidotic, but the renal compensation for his long-standing CO_2 retention will have generated a higher than normal bicarbonate and he will have a base excess in his 'normal' state. If he becomes ill enough, he could well develop a metabolic acidosis (because of anaerobic metabolism etc.) and his acid-base status will be very complicated.

V.53 TFFFF

Another tricky clinical question. Look at ALL the points; they must ALL fit. This is a false situation; you never have to make diagnoses on this type of half-information — but you're stuck with it!

B Why cyanosed?
C Epigastric pain radiating through to the back is an uncommon presentation of myocardial infarction, plus absent bowel sounds must make it more unlikely.
D,E Why cyanosed?

V.54 TFTFT

B,D Both are relatively unlikely to respond well.

V.55 TFFFF

B,C,E These are contra-indications for a shunt.
D A prophylactic shunt will not increase life expectancy, even in the otherwise fit young patient.

V.56 TFTFF

A This is apparently a feature of early perforation.
B Pain can be anywhere, but is likely to be central.
C Air under the diaphragm will give shoulder pain.
D No — this is a distinguishing feature from acute pancreatitis.
E Why should there be haemodilution? Later there will be haemoconcentration.

V.57 TFFTT

B Vomiting is usually early but not persistent.
C Pyrexia and tachycardia do not occur early, and the pyrexia is not usually extreme.
E The risk of perforation, and the mortality, are both much greater in babies.

V.58 TFFTT

A The metabolic alkalosis reduces the ionized calcium.
B Not in chronic obstruction.
C The only mechanism might be supine hypotension due to caval compression: not really!

V.59 TTTFT

B The median and ulnar nerves can be damaged, but damage is uncommon.

D Loss of the radial pulse is an indication for strict observation, but surgery is not needed, provided that the circulation is adequate.

V.60 FTTFF

A Straining is no help: the patient must just wait.

D An intravenous pyelogram is performed UNLESS there is renal failure.

E Only if passing and then removing the catheter fails to restore normal micturition.

Paper VI Questions

VI.1 If ventilation is impossible after apparently successful intubation, one should think of:

- **A** kinking of the endotracheal tube as it passes over the back of the tongue
- **B** oesophageal intubation
- **C** right main bronchial intubation
- **D** herniated cuff
- **E** severe bronchospasm.

VI.2 Depending on the cause, appropriate treatment of intra-operative hypotension includes:

- **A** dopamine
- **B** sodium bicarbonate
- **C** phentolamine
- **D** ephedrine
- **E** ergometrine.

VI.3 Immediate treatment of a post-operative thyrotoxic crisis includes:

- **A** heavy sedation
- **B** chlorpromazine
- **C** steroids
- **D** propranolol
- **E** intravenous calcium gluconate.

VI.4 In a 5-year-old child who is bleeding after elective adenotonsillectomy:

- **A** shock is unlikely to be severe
- **B** sedation should be avoided to minimize cardiovascular depression
- **C** the patient's serum should be grouped and saved prior to induction
- **D** gaseous induction is preferable
- **E** anaesthesia should be induced in the supine position to allow rapid endotracheal intubation.

VI.5 In blind-nasal intubation:

A carbon dioxide may be added to the inspired gas mixture to facilitate intubation
B a single dose of propanidid may produce sufficient hyperventilation for the technique
C the tube may pass into the oesophagus if the neck is excessively flexed
D mucosal lacerative over the arch of the atlas is a common cause of bleeding
E thiopentone is contra-indicated as an induction agent.

VI.6 In men over 50 years of age, the statistical probability of a myocardial infarction occurring in the post-operative period is:

A decreased if a high inspired oxygen concentration is used during anaesthesia
B increased if there is a history of myocardial infarction
C increased by prolongation of surgery
D increased with pre-operative evidence of ST segment depression
E increased with pre-operative history of angina.

VI.7 Awareness during anaesthesia:

A is only a problem in unpremedicated patients
B is recognized by constriction of the pupil
C is associated with tachycardia and production of tears
D is prevented in most patients by 0.5% halothane
E is associated with an altered sensation of pain.

VI.8 Pre-operative management of a jaundiced patient about to undergo diagnostic laparotomy should include:

A a full clotting screen
B pre-operative mannitol therapy
C prophylactic antibiotics
D intravenous vitamin K
E histamine (H_2) receptor antagonist therapy.

VI.9 A patient presenting for elective hysterectomy is found to have a haemoglobin concentration of 7 g/dl. You should:

A delay surgery and transfuse the patient with packed cells
B proceed with anaesthesia and surgery, transfusing the patient with whole blood intra-operatively
C administer spinal anaesthesia
D proceed with anaesthesia, but set up a dextran infusion
E proceed with anaesthesia using a high oxygen concentration.

VI.10 Suitable sedative techniques for use in intensive care include:

A thiopentone infusion
B midazolam infusion
C phenoperidine
D etomidate infusion
E lytic cocktail.

VI.11 Late complications of nasotracheal intubation include:

A deafness
B maxillary abscess
C sloughing of the pharyngeal mucosa
D necrosis of alar cartilage
E transient cranial mononeuropathy of left recurrent laryngeal nerve.

VI.12 Elective hypotension in neurosurgery:

A is satisfactorily achieved with halothane and IPPV
B is contra-indicated in surgery for intracranial aneurysm
C affects autoregulation of the cerebral circulation
D is associated with a reduction in cerebral oxygenation
E increases the risk of air embolism.

VI.13 Appropriate treatment of air embolism occurring during posterior fossa surgery includes:

A jugular compression
B increasing the mean intrathoracic pressure
C aspiration via a central venous catheter
D a mannitol infusion
E turning the patient onto the left side, head down.

VI.14 Appropriate prophylaxis against the acid-aspiration syndrome includes:

A mist. magnesium trisilicate
B metoclopramide
C hydrocortisone
D pre-operative passage of a nasogastric tube
E sodium citrate.

VI.15 A 35-year-old primigravida is induced at 37 weeks because of pre-eclampsia. She is complaining of tingling in her fingers but is otherwise asymptomatic. The following would be reasons for avoiding epidural analgesia:

A a diastolic blood pressure above 120 mm Hg
B persistent fetal tachycardia
C signs of disordered blood clotting
D heavy proteinuria
E refusal by the patient.

VI.16 Appropriate treatment in a patient thought to have suffered an amniotic fluid embolus includes:

A blood transfusion
B heparin
C ephedrine
D steroids
E salbutamol.

VI.17 A healthy 6-week-old baby presents with pyloric stenosis and requires general anaesthesia for Ramstedt's operation. A suitable anaesthetic technique includes:

A intravenous induction with thiopentone
B intubation under neuromuscular blockade with alcuronium
C 0.1 mg atropine as premedication
D intravenous fluid therapy with sodium chloride
E spontaneous ventilation with oxygen and halothane.

VI.18 The following are true of thiopentone:

A the sympathetic stimulation produced prevents severe hypotension
B hypotension commonly occurs due to vasodilation
C extravascular injection may produce cutaneous sloughing
D porphyria may be precipitated
E it is the agent of choice in asthmatics.

VI.19 Nitrous oxide:

A does not combine with haemoglobin
B produces increased tension in a pneumothorax
C may induce bone marrow aplasia
D is partially metabolized in the liver
E induces diffusion hypoxia at the termination of anaesthesia.

VI.20 Features of anaesthesia with trichloroethylene include:

A rapid induction of anaesthesia
B tachypnoea
C adequate relaxation
D adequate analgesia
E cardiac dysrhythmias.

VI.21 In the detection of abnormal serum cholinesterase:

A dibucaine inhibits serum cholinesterase
B 97% of the population possess the normal enzyme
C in patients homozygous for the abnormal enzyme, the dibucaine number is in excess of 80%
D in the 3% of patients who are heterozygous for the abnormal enzyme, the dibucaine number is approximately 60%
E fluoride is used as an alternative enzyme inhibitor.

VI.22 Bronchospasm complicating anaesthesia is likely to be associated with:

A the use of suxamethonium
B induction with etomidate
C fluid replacement with dextran
D rapid intravenous injection of metoclopramide
E blood transfusion.

VI.23 After pneumonectomy:

A a single chest drain is commonly used
B chest drainage must be allowed to bubble freely
C a Maxwell box may be used to centralize the mediastinum
D tension pneumothorax is a common cause of hypotension
E there is often surgical emphysema

VI.24 The following are true of the muscles of the pharynx:

A the superior constrictor is stylopharyngeus
B cricopharyngeus is the inferior part of the lower constrictor and is composed of transverse fibres
C functionally cricopharyngeus is a sphincter
D pharyngeal pouches tend to occur anteriorly through the lower constrictor
E the constrictor muscles are supplied by nerve fibres from the vagus and glossopharyngeal nerves.

VI.25 The cephalic vein:

A is one of the major deep veins of the upper limb
B communicates with the basilic vein via the median cubital vein
C at the elbow lies between brachoradialis and biceps
D in the upper arm lies in the delto-pectoral groove
E drains directly into the axillary vein.

VI.26 Block of the brachial plexus by the supraclavicular route:

- **A** aims to deposit local anaesthetic solution around the trunks as they emerge from beneath the first rib
- **B** a total of 15 ml 2% lignocaine with adrenaline should be sufficient
- **C** technique should not include a nerve stimulator because of the danger of pleural burns
- **D** unlike axillary block, it will allow placement of an upper arm tourniquet
- **E** occasionally fails properly to anaesthetize the palmar skin.

VI.27 The dura mater:

- **A** is a double membrane extending from within the cranium to the filum terminale
- **B** is attached above to the edges of the foramen magnum
- **C** is attached posteriorly by the posterior longitudinal ligament
- **D** encloses the dural sac down to the level of approximately the second sacral segment
- **E** at spinal level is lined by the arachnoid mater.

VI.28 The following are true of nerves supplying extra-ocular muscles:

- **A** an oculomotor palsy results in loss of the accommodation reflex
- **B** an oculomotor palsy results in enophthalmos and ptosis
- **C** a trochlear (IV) palsy results in diplopia on looking down and out
- **D** a sixth nerve (abducent) palsy results in a divergent squint
- **E** the sixth nerve is particularly liable to damage because it has a thin connective tissue sheath.

VI.29 The glossopharyngeal nerve:

- **A** supplies all pharyngeal sensation except for the tonsil
- **B** supplies sensation to the posterior third of the tongue
- **C** passes through the jugular foramen
- **D** supplies fibres to the otic ganglion
- **E** carries afferent information from the carotid sinus and carotid body.

VI.30 The lateral popliteal (common peroneal) nerve:

- **A** subserves sensation on the dorsum of the foot via the musculocutaneous (superficial peroneal) nerve
- **B** subserves sensation over the whole of the dorsum of the foot
- **C** is a sensory nerve
- **D** supplies the skin over a variable area of the lateral lower leg
- **E** ends as the anterior tibial and medial calcaneal nerves.

VI.31 Cervical plexus block:

- **A** is effective with about 4 ml of 1.5% lignocaine at the transverse processes of C3–5
- **B** if performed bilaterally, and combined with a light general anaesthetic, gives a good, bloodless field for thyroidectomy
- **C** is likely to give a Horner's syndrome
- **D** is best performed avoiding solutions containing adrenaline
- **E** dural puncture is a recognized complication.

VI.32 Hypokalaemia is likely to be associated with:

- **A** diarrhoea
- **B** excess mineralocorticoid secretion
- **C** triamterene administration
- **D** metabolic alkalosis
- **E** uretero-colic anastamosis.

VI.33 In the electrocardiogram:

- **A** the QT interval varies with the blood calcium
- **B** low potassium is associated with a prolonged QT interval
- **C** low potassium is accompanied by ST depression
- **D** biphasic P-waves occur with very high potassium levels
- **E** the PR interval is short in Wolff-Parkinson-White syndrome.

VI.34 Common causes of pericarditis include:

- **A** viral infection
- **B** acute myocardial infarction
- **C** pulmonary embolism
- **D** tuberculosis
- **E** uraemia.

VI.35 Causes of atrial fibrillation include:

- **A** thyrotoxicosis
- **B** rheumatic heart disease
- **C** cardiomyopathy
- **D** hypertension
- **E** atropine administration.

VI.36 The maintenance dose of digoxin should be reduced in:

- **A** thyrotoxicosis
- **B** myocardial infarction
- **C** impaired renal function
- **D** cardiopulmonary bypass
- **E** the elderly.

VI.37 In malignant hypertension, there is an increased likelihood of:

- **A** cerebral haemorrhage
- **B** renal failure
- **C** congestive cardiac failure
- **D** left ventricular failure
- **E** pulmonary hypertension.

VI.38 A diastolic cardiac murmur is associated with:

- **A** mitral incompetence
- **B** increased atrioventricular flow occurring in a patient with a patient VSD
- **C** aortic regurgitation
- **D** atrioseptal defect
- **E** patent ductus arteriosus.

VI.39 Excessively high glucocorticoid levels occur in or cause:

- **A** dehydration
- **B** hypertension
- **C** muscle weakness
- **D** potassium depletion
- **E** osteoporosis.

VI.40 Likely symptoms in a patient suffering from hypothyroidism include:

- **A** prolongation of opiate metabolism
- **B** hypoglycaemia
- **C** hypothermia
- **D** positive Trousseau's sign
- **E** prolonged response to non-depolarizing neuromuscular blocking drugs.

VI.41 Hypothermia:

- **A** complicates chlorpromazine therapy
- **B** occurs in acute pancreatitis
- **C** is best treated by rapid, active rewarming
- **D** occurs in myxoedema
- **E** is likely to occur intra-operatively at the extremes of age.

VI.42 The following are true of Crohn's disease:

- **A** it affects predominantly females
- **B** it affects only the terminal portion of the ileum
- **C** it is more likely than ulcerative colitis to lead to fistulae
- **D** it is associated with uveitis
- **E** sufferers have auto-antibodies.

VI.43 Causes of intestinal malabsorption include:

- **A** coeliac disease
- **B** hyperparathyroidism
- **C** diabetes mellitus
- **D** carcinoid syndrome
- **E** tropical sprue.

VI.44 The following occur in haemophilia:

- **A** haemarthrosis
- **B** prolonged bleeding time
- **C** prolonged partial thromboplastin time
- **D** impaired clot retraction
- **E** haemorrhagic skin rash.

VI.45 Dystrophia myotonica:

- **A** is a primary disorder of the myoneural junction
- **B** is associated with cataract formation
- **C** is associated with gonadal atrophy
- **D** only occurs in males
- **E** is associated with limb weakness.

VI.46 Myasthenia gravis:

- **A** disseminated lupus erythematosus is an association
- **B** 15% will have a thymoma
- **C** ophthalmoplegia alone is a presentation
- **D** blood gases are a good guide to ventilatory function
- **E** pyridostigmine is better than neostigmine because overdose does not cause a depolarization block.

VI.47 The following statements concerning a patient on oral hypoglycaemic drugs are true:

- **A** chlorpropamide has a half-life of 36 hours
- **B** phenformin increases lactic acid production
- **C** glibenclamide stimulates anaerobic metabolism
- **D** the duration of action of glibenclamide is less than six hours
- **E** hypoglycaemia may be precipitated by concomitant administration of intravenous cephalosporin antibiotics.

VI.48 Common findings in a patient with acute renal failure include:

- **A** metabolic acidosis
- **B** hyperkalaemia
- **C** anaemia
- **D** decreased circulating fluid volume
- **E** cerebral oedema.

VI.49 In polycystic disease of the kidney:

A inheritance is an autosomal dominant
B presentation is usually in middle adult life
C pyelonephritis is a common complication
D hypertension is a common complication
E life expectancy is little reduced if the patients follow a renal diet.

VI.50 A reduction in total lung compliance is commonly associated with:

A left ventricular failure
B emphysema
C kyphoscoliosis
D pulmonary fibrosis
E asthma.

VI.51 Endocrine syndromes associated with primary bronchogenic carcinoma include:

A inappropriate ADH secretion
B hyperglycaemia
C thyrotoxicosis
D oedema, polyuria and weakness
E carcinoid syndrome.

VI.52 A 35-year-old woman with a history of asthma is brought into casualty acutely dyspnoeic. She usually uses salbutamol and cromoglycate inhalers and has been on prednisolone 5 mg daily for two months:

A now she is in hospital, steroids should be discontinued
B if her $PaCO_2$ is 4 kPa, it is probably safe not to start IPPV immediately
C she should not be given more than 35% O_2 by mask
D she should lie down to make her breathing easier
E she will have a prolonged inspiratory time.

VI.53 A 58-year-old man is brought into casualty with 35% burns, having had a gas stove explode in his face. He is conscious, in pain, and he is distressed:

A opiates should be avoided
B an intravenous infusion of 5% dextrose should be started immediately
C if he needs an anaesthetic, he must not be given suxamethonium
D arterial blood should be taken for gas analysis
E serial haematocrit measurement is a good aid to fluid replacement.

VI.54 Indications for splenectomy include:

- **A** myelofibrosis
- **B** idiopathic thrombocytopenic purpura
- **C** spontaneous rupture due to infectious mononucleosis
- **D** Hodgkin's disease
- **E** hereditary spherocytosis.

VI.55 The following are true of traumatic rupture of the spleen:

- **A** it is more likely to occur in infectious mononucleosis
- **B** it is more likely in malaria
- **C** the abdomen is soft, provided other viscera are not injured
- **D** rupture delayed more than 14 days is well-recognized
- **E** radiological signs include obliteration of the psoas shadow.

VI.56 A 5-year-old child is suspected of having acute appendicitis. The following are likely to confirm this diagnosis:

- **A** a rectal temperature of 40°C
- **B** bronchial breathing at the right lung base
- **C** urinary sample with five white cells per high-powered field
- **D** pain in the right iliac fossa when pressing on the left of the abdomen
- **E** diarrhoea the previous evening.

VI.57 The following are true of rupture of the oesophagus:

- **A** the patient is usually surprisingly well
- **B** prognosis is better in spontaneous rupture than rupture following instrumentation
- **C** surgical emphysema is a common sign
- **D** the need for surgical repair is extremely urgent
- **E** a barium swallow may be helpful if there is doubt in diagnosis.

VI.58 Likely complications of laparoscopy include:

- **A** hypotension
- **B** regurgitation
- **C** shoulder pain
- **D** gas embolism
- **E** deep venous thrombosis.

VI.59 Following the prolapse of an intervertebral disc:

- **A** at L4–5 there will be weakness of ankle dorsiflexion
- **B** at L4–5 the ankle jerk will be preserved
- **C** at L5–S1 there will be pain in the calf
- **D** bladder symptoms are an indication for urgent surgery
- **E** myelography should be performed before surgery.

VI.60 The use of large quantities of isotonic non-electrolyte-containing solutions for irrigation during prolonged transurethral prostatic resection results in:

A hyponatraemia
B haemolysis
C haemodilution
D hyperkalaemia
E hypoglycaemia.

Paper VI Answers

VI.1 **TTFTT**

C Ventilation is far from impossible in this situation!

VI.2 **TTFTF**

A If the problem is myocardial depression.
B If acidosis is depressing the myocardium.
C Phentolamine is an alpha-blocker which will induce vasodilation.
D Particularly when caused by spinal or epidural blockade.
E Used as an oxytocic and not for its vasoconstricting action.

VI.3 **TTTTF**

The word 'immediate' is included.
V.40 was similar.

A,B,C,D All produce symptomatic improvement.
E For tetany after parathyroidectomy.

VI.4 **FFFTF**

Compare with I.4.

A Patients still bleed to death after tonsillectomy.
B Initial treatment is sedation to give the haemorrhage a chance to stop.
C Blood must be cross-matched.
D This is the textbook answer, although an experienced anaesthetist might choose a careful intravenous induction, depending on the particular circumstances.
E On the left side to minimize the risks of aspiration of blood.

VI.5 TTTFF

B Propanidid — in Cremophor — has been withdrawn.

D It occurs, but is not a COMMON cause. The commonest cause is minor trauma in the nasal passages.

E Not so, provided intubation is not attempted on thiopentone alone.

VI.6 FTFTT

A High inspired oxygen concentrations do not affect the probability unless they are necessary to maintain an adequate pO_2, i.e. in seriously ill patients only.

C Pulmonary problems, yes, but not myocardial infarction.

VI.7 FFTTF

A May still occur, although amnesia may prevent recall.

B Dilation usually.

E Not necessarily — pain may still occur.

VI.8 TTTTF

E No real reason why — the patient may be obstructed, but does not necessarily have a high gastric acid.

VI.9 TFFFF

B–E If a patient for elective surgery is severely anaemic, correct treatment is to postpone surgery and treat the anaemia. No anaesthetic technique is particularly appropriate, nor will any of the alternatives except the first improve tissue oxygenation markedly.

VI.10 TTTFT

A,B,C,E All these are used in various situations, particularly severe head injuries.

D Etomidate is no longer recommended because of the associated adrenocortical suppression.

VI.11 TTTTT

E Sounds wonderful and is true, though rather rare!

VI.12 FFTTF

A Not satisfactory, because the concentration of halothane needed would increase cerebral blood flow.

D Not when vasodilation is used.

E Doesn't affect venous pressure.

VI.13 TTTFT

D Mannitol may be used if cerebral swelling occurs as a result of air embolism, but it is not a treatment for the condition.

VI.14 TTFFT

C Not a prophylactic measure.

D A nasogastric tube makes the patient more likely to vomit, probably renders the cardia incompetent and is not guaranteed to empty the stomach.

VI.15 FFTFT

Epidural analgesia is recommended in pre-eclampsia, and early in labour rather than late. In severe pre-eclampsia (**A**), the BP may not be reduced by the technique, because it is a disease of the small vessels, but that is not a reason for avoidance.

B,D Irrelevant.

E The patient must always be considered — though one can try to persuade!

VI.16 TTTTT

B A coagulopathy is likely: heparin may help, though it is a good idea to involve the haematologists because clotting disorders can be complex and tend to change character rapidly.

VI.17 TFTTT

A 6-week-old baby will probably be a bit too vigorous for an awake intubation.

B Intubation in the face of pyloric obstruction would be better carried out using suxamethonium.

E Gaseous induction should include cricoid pressure.

VI.18 FTTTF

A Peripheral vasodilator, unrelated to sympathetic effects.

A,B THESE ARE MUTUALLY EXCLUSIVE.

E Not so — because of laryngeal sensitization and bronchospasm. Thiopentone anaphylaxis is IgE mediated.

VI.19 TTTFT

VI.20 FTFTT

A A soluble agent that has a slow induction.

C No relaxant properties.

VI.21 TTFTT

C It is easy to get this the wrong way around. Homozygous patients possess only abnormal enzyme. This is dibucaine-resistant, so that inhibition, at 16–20%, is less than normal, which is 80%.

D This is true: you have to know both figures are correct.

VI.22 TFTFT

A Suxamethonium does cause histamine release.

B Etomidate alone is not commonly associated with bronchospasm.

C,E Dextran solutions and blood products can cause allergic reactions.

D Metoclopramide rarely produces hypersensitivity.

VI.23 TFTFF

B Clamped to prevent mediastinal movement.

C An external device used to regulate the volume of air in the chest and ensure that the mediastinum remains central.

D Not a common cause, provided the drain is clamped.

E Rarely present.

VI.24 TTTFF

B,C The tranverse fibres form a sphincter.

D Posterolaterally between the functionally different upper and lower fibres.

E Vagal and accessory fibres.

VI.25 FTTTT

A It is a superficial vein: most of the venous drainage of the arm is through superficial veins.

D A site for percutaneous puncture and particularly for direct cut-down.

VI.26 FFFFT

A As they CROSS the first rib.

B Too small a volume: 30–40 ml 1–2% lignocaine with adrenaline.

C Using a stimulator improves the success rate: the comment about pleural burns is a red herring.

D Neither route guarantees analgesia of the inner aspect of the upper arm.

E The median nerve (middle trunk, C7) sometimes escapes.

VI.27 FTFTT

A It is double only inside the cranium, the two layers enclosing the cerebral sinuses.

C It is attached ANTERIORLY TO the posterior longitudinal ligament.

VI.28 TFTTF

A The pupillary constrictor is paralysed.

B Ptosis only; enophthalmos and ptosis occur in a Horner's (SNS paralysis).

E NO — it is vulnerable because of its long course.

VI.29 FTTTT

A Including the tonsil.

D PNS fibres via the lesser superficial petrosal nerve.

VI.30 TTFTF

B,E The anterior tibial is also a branch of the lateral popliteal. The medial calcaneal is a cutaneous branch of the posterior tibial that supplies the heel.

C It is a mixed nerve: it contains sensory and motor fibres. Thus to describe it as a sensory nerve, even though it contains sensory fibres, is incorrect.

VI.31 TFTTT

This is tiger country so: avoid adrenaline (**D**), aspirate carefully (**D, E**); and bilateral block (**B**) should not be undertaken lightly (it can result in bilateral phrenic paralysis).

VI.32 TTFTT

C Triamterene is an aldosterone antagonist, tending to conserve potassium at the expense of sodium.

E Urine in the colon decreases transit time and therefore increases potassium excretion.

VI.33 TTTTT

VI.34 TTFFT

C,D The question includes the word 'commonly' and questions should be assumed to apply to practice in the Western world unless stated otherwise.

VI.35 TTTTF

E Not associated with atrial fibrillation — although heart rate is increased, sinus rhythm is maintained and may even revert spontaneously in a patient with relatively slow AF.

VI.36 FFTTT

B It may be deleterious to reduce the dose.

D Digoxin is usually stopped pre-operatively because defibrillation of a digitalized heart is much less effective.

VI.37 TTFTF

C,E In malignant hypertension, the cardiac lesions are left-sided, resulting in left ventricular hypertrophy etc.

VI.38 FTTFF

A Mitral incompetence causes a systolic murmur, stenosis a diastolic one.

E Not a distolic murmur, but a continuous machinery murmur.

VI.39 FTTTT

A They usually cause fluid retention and oedema.

B Cushing's syndrome.

B–E May be of endogenous or iatrogenic causation.

VI.40 TTTFT

D This occurs in hypoparathyroidism, not hypothyroidism.

VI.41 TFFTT

A Because of vasodilation.

B Shock yes, but not hypothermia specifically.

C Rapid, active rewarming may produce cardiac dysrhythmias and even cardiac arrest.

VI.42 FFTFF

A There is no sex difference in Crohn's disease.

B Although commonest here, it can affect any part of the gastro-intestinal tract.

D There may occasionally be iritis.

E Not yet demonstrated.

VI.43 TFTTT

B Hypo- but not hyperparathyroidism.

VI.44 TTFFF

C This is a test of the intrinsic pathway and of the prothrombin-dependent factors.

D Clot retraction is a platelet-dependent effect.

E Skin rashes are not a feature of haemophilia.

VI.45 FTTTT

A Dystrophia myotonica is a disorder of the muscle fibres themselves, not the myoneural junction.

VI.46 TTTFF

C In some patients with ophthalmoplegia the disease never progresses.

D Changes in blood gases are a late result of ventilatory failure in myaesthenia.

E Pyridostigmine is longer-acting.

VI.47 TTFFF

C Only a side-effect of the diguanide oral hypoglycaemics.

D 12–16 hours.

E Sounds good, but is a red herring!

VI.48 TTTFT

D Circulating fluid volume will be normal or increased.

VI.49 TTTTF

E Life expectancy is reduced in polycystic disease of the kidneys.

VI.50 TFTTF

B Increased in emphysema.
E Certainly not reduced in asthma, though resistance is much increased.

VI.51 TFTTT

B Hypo-rather than hyperglycaemia.
D Due to ectopic ACTH production.

VI.52 FTFFF

A The dose of steroids may have to be increased.
B A NORMAL pCO_2 in acute asthma is a sign that IPPV may be needed.
C She should be given humidified oxygen in high concentration.
D Breathing is likely to be easier sitting up.
E Prolonged expiratory time.

VI.53 FFFTT

A Opiates can be given with care.
B Plasma or saline, certainly not dextrose.
C If immediately after the incident, suxamethonium can be used. Classically the problem of excess rise in plasma K^+ with suxamethonium occurs at 3–5 weeks.

VI.54 TTTTT

B Removing the spleen in ITP helps to preserve the platelets.

D Splenectomy is frequently part of a staging laparotomy in lymphomas.

VI.55 TTFTT

C Over half the patients show rigidity.

D Late delayed rupture is not common, but is well-recognized.

VI.56 TFFTF

The important words are 'symptoms LIKELY TO CONFIRM the diagnosis'.

B,C,E All these would, if anything, make the diagnosis doubtful.

VI.57 FFTTF

A,B They are usually in great distress, especially after spontaneous rupture. This usually follows vomiting, and gastric contents in the mediastinum will make the patient very ill.

E Lipiodol yes, barium no — it is an irritant to the mediastinal tissues.

VI.58 TTTFF

Beware of the inclusion of the word 'likely'.

D,E Both have been reported, but are they LIKELY to occur, in your experience?

VI.59 TTTTT

All of these are true.

VI.60 TFTFT

A,C,E Dilutional, due to absorption of isotonic fluid containing no electrolytes.

B Not with isotonic fluid.

D Dilution would produce hypokalaemia.

Paper VII Questions

VII.1 Features of rhematoid arthritis likely to influence anaesthetic management when a patient is undergoing coincidental surgery include:

A stridor
B amyloidosis of the kidney
C pulmonary fibrosis
D erosion of the odontoid peg
E anaemia.

VII.2 A hypertensive patient, receiving a diuretic and propranolol (80 mg three times a day), presenting for anaesthesia for major gastric surgery should:

A have his propranolol replaced by methyldopa pre-operatively
B have a pre-operative ECG
C continue to receive his antihypertensive therapy up to the time of operation
D receive intravenous propranolol during surgery
E only receive 5 ml/kg/hour crystalloid replacement to avoid fluid overload.

VII.3 Appropriate pre-operative therapy in a patient with hyperthyroidism controlled on propranolol includes:

A reduce propranolol and discontinue on the evening prior to operation
B pre-operative corticosteroid cover
C substitution of carbimazole for propranolol immediately pre-operatively
D addition of pre-operative potassium iodide
E peri-operative maintenance of propranolol therapy.

VII.4 In a patient presenting with laryngeal carcinoma for elective laryngectomy:

A stridor is uncommon
B operative resection should be preceded by tracheostomy under local anaesthesia if respiratory obstruction is present
C opiate premedication should not be used because of the risk of respiratory depression
D hypotension and cardiac arrythmias occur during mobilization of the larynx
E post-operative disturbances of calcium metabolism are a recognized complication.

VII.5 Concerning gases and cylinders:

A the working pressure of a modern anaesthetic machine is 60 lb/sq in
B the filling ratio of a nitrous oxide cylinder is 0.69
C blue cylinders contain liquid nitrous oxide
D the pressure of a full oxygen cylinder is about 2000 lb/sq in
E the pressure of a full cylinder of nitrous oxide is 900 lb/sq in.

VII.6 Malignant hyperpyrexia:

A develops intra-operatively without any prodromal symptoms or signs
B is precipitated by suxamethonium
C requires monitoring of body temperature for a diagnosis to be made
D is accompanied by shivering in the anaesthetized patient
E is best treated with intravenous procaine and regional hypothermia.

VII.7 Opiate premedication;

A is given for its vagotonic effect
B may be given orally
C is contra-indicated in children
D slows gastric emptying
E promotes hepatic clearance of anaesthetic agents.

VII.8 The use of nitrous oxide is contra-indicated in anaesthesia for

A pneumo-encephalography
B large bowel resection
C bronchopleural fistula
D posterior fossa surgery
E cystic pulmonary disease.

VII.9 Decompression sickness:

A is associated with avascular necrosis of bone
B is due to an alveolar oxygen deficit
C is cured by breathing a mixture of oxygen and helium
D occurs up to four hours after the initial drop in pressure
E is avoided if nitrogen is included in the inspired gas mixture.

VII.10 Likely complications of infraclavicular subclavian venous cannulation include:

A recurrent laryngeal nerve palsy
B air embolism
C pneumothorax
D phrenic nerve palsy
E haemopericardium.

VII.11 Characteristic direct features of overdosage of a tricyclic antidepressant include:

A convulsions
B metabolic acidosis
C cardiac arrhythmias
D hypothermia
E respiratory alkalosis.

VII.12 Post-operative cerebral vasospasm occurring in a patient with a subarachnoid haemorrhage:

A is safe, provided that the aneurysm has been clipped successfully
B is treated with intravenous infusion of low molecular weight dextran
C increases the risk of a subsequent haemorrhage
D is an absolute indication for post-operative ventilation
E presents as a hemiplegia.

VII.13 Intracranial pressure is reduced by:

A intravenous urea
B halothane
C phenytoin
D barbiturates
E suxamethonium.

VII.14 Pre-anaesthetic antacid therapy for Caesarian section may be satisfactorily achieved with:

A sodium citrate
B glycopyrollate
C mist. magnesium trisilicate
D potassium borate
E Epsom salts.

VII.15 Acute inversion of the uterus following delivery causes:

A cyanosis
B hypotension
C bradycardia
D hypofibrinogenaemia
E severe haemorrhage.

VII.16 Post-partum shock is associated with:

A amniotic fluid embolism
B acute inversion of the uterus
C eclampsia
D disseminated intravascular coagulation
E placenta praevia.

VII.17 A 6-month-old infant of Greek parents presents with a one-week history of malaise and anorexia. Examination reveals multiple bruising on the limbs and scalp, inflamed and swollen gums, a rectal temperature of 38°C, and a painful left leg held in flexion. Likely diagnoses include:

A scurvy
B osteomyelitis and septicaemia
C haemophilia
D child abuse
E idiopathic thrombocytopaenia.

VII.18 Skin blood flow is:

A increased by halothane anaesthesia
B increased in sympathetic activity
C unchanged in methoxyflurane anaesthesia
D decreased in barbiturate anaesthesia
E unchanged in cardiogenic shock.

VII.19 Intraoperative analgesia in man is satisfactorily achieved with:

A phenoperidine
B levorphanol
C etorphine
D ketamine
E indoramin.

VII.20 Drugs which can safely be used in a patient with acute intermittent porphyria include:

A pethidine
B chlorpromazine
C phenylbutazone
D methohexitone
E phenytoin.

VII.21 Suxamethonium therapy causes clinically significant elevation of serum potassium concentrations in patients suffering from:

A pseudohypertrophic muscular dystrophy
B uraemia
C tetanus
D paraplegia
E diabetes mellitus.

VII.22 A patient presenting for abdominal surgery gives a history of chronic obstructive airways disease and is dyspnoeic at rest. Useful tests to establish his fitness for anaesthesia include:

A arterial blood gases
B nitrogen washout
C ventilatory response to breathing 100% oxygen
D FEV_1 and FVC
E carbon monoxide transfer factor.

VII.23 In a patient with a bronchopleural fistula, induction of anaesthesia must include:

A awake intubation
B endobronchial intubation
C the use of non-depolarizing neuromuscular blocking drugs
D the pre-operative insertion of a patent chest drain
E the avoidance of nitrous oxide.

VII.24 In the larynx and associated structures:

A the vocal cord is attached posteriorly via the vocal process to the arytenoid cartilage
B the cricoid cartilage articulates below with the thyroid cartilage and above with the arytenoids
C the cricothyroid ligament is an anterior thickening of the cricovocal membrane
D the hyoid bone is at the level of the third cervical vertebra
E the isthmus of the thyroid gland is just below the inferior border of the thyroid cartilage.

VII.25 The following complications may follow unilateral supraclavicular block of the brachial plexus:

A respiratory paralysis because of phrenic blockade
B puncture of the subclavian artery
C pneumothorax
D dural puncture
E epileptiform convulsions.

VII.26 The basilic vein:

A is the continuation of the superficial palmar venous arch
B ascends initially on the posterior ulnar aspect of the forearm
C is related to the medial cutaneous nerve of forearm
D lies medial to biceps in the upper arm
E is a better catheterization route than the cephalic vein because it does not perforate the deep fascia.

VII.27 The extradural space;

A is contiguous with the pleural cavity
B extends from the 4th ventricle to the sacral hiatus
C contains fat, arteries and veins but no lymphatic vessels
D has valveless veins that provide a direct connection between the pelvic and cerebral veins
E provides a recirculation pathway for extravasated cerebrospinal fluid.

VII.28 The trigeminal nerve:

A is the fifth and largest cranial nerve
B provides sensation to the face and most of the scalp
C provides somatic sensation to the eyeball
D provides sensation to the anterior two-thirds of the buccal mucosa, hard palate and tongue
E supplies the muscles of mastication.

VII.29 The following are true of the facial nerve:

A it supplies salivary secretomotor fibres
B it supplies lacrimal secretomotor fibres
C an intracranial lesion usually results in involvement of the auditory nerve as well
D compression by an acoustic neuroma will not cause paralysis of the forehead
E it traverses the eardrum.

VII.30 An ankle block requires the application of local anaesthetic to:

A the posterior tibial nerve between the Achilles tendon and the medial malleolus
B the sural nerve between the Achilles tendon and the lateral malleolus
C the anterior tibial nerve anteriorly midway between the malleoli
D the musculocutaneous nerve by subcutaneous injection from the front of the tibia to the lateral malleolus
E the saphenous nerve just above the medial malleolus.

VII.31 Raised plasma bicarbonate is associated with:

A renal failure
B persistent vomiting
C diabetes insipidus
D rheumatoid arthritis
E hepatic coma.

VII.32 Serum electrolyte measurements of Na^+ 125 and K^+ 6.2 mmol/l are consistent with a diagnosis of;

- **A** acute renal failure
- **B** hypopituitarism
- **C** Addison's disease
- **D** primary hyperaldersteronism
- **E** Cushing's disease.

VII.33 Suitable methods for the treatment of paroxysmal atrial tachycardia include:

- **A** carotid sinus massage
- **B** disopyramide
- **C** synchronized DC defibrillation
- **D** eyeball pressure
- **E** intravenous methoxamine.

VII.34 Causes of right bundle branch block include:

- **A** pulmonary embolism
- **B** myxoedema
- **C** myocardial ischaemia
- **D** myotonia congenita
- **E** atrial septal defect.

VII.35 Digitalis has the following effects on the ECG:

- **A** decreased R–R interval
- **B** shortened Q–T interval
- **C** first-degree heart block
- **D** prominent U-waves
- **E** the effects are proportional to the efficacy of treatment.

VII.36 Following acute myocardial infarction, appropriate treatment for multifocal ventricular extrasystoles occurring at a rate of 10 per minute in a patient in sinus rhythm at 80 beats per minute and with a blood pressure of 110/70 includes:

- **A** atropine 500 μg intravenously
- **B** propranolol 1 mg intravenously
- **C** controlled 28% oxygen therapy
- **D** lignocaine 100 mg intravenously
- **E** verapamil 5 mg intravenously.

VII.37 A low, fixed cardiac output occurs in:

- **A** aortic stenosis
- **B** constrictive pericarditis
- **C** mitral stenosis
- **D** cor pulmonale
- **E** digoxin toxicity

VII.38 A 68-year-old man, a known hypertensive taking metoprolol, is admitted to casualty with central chest pain. He is pale and sweaty and has a blood pressure of 70/50. The following are true:

- **A** 80 mg of intravenous frusemide should be given
- **B** intravenous lignocaine is reasonable treatment for multiple ventricular ectopic beats
- **C** verapamil is reasonable treatment for atrial fibrillation
- **D** a high central venous pressure indicates poor left ventricular function
- **E** he should be given a high concentration of oxygen by mask.

VII.39 The following are true of carcinoid syndrome:

- **A** the primary is commonly jejunal or ileal
- **B** the clinical syndrome occurs when the primary exceeds about 100 g
- **C** diarrhoea occurs
- **D** asthmatic attacks occur
- **E** tricuspid stenosis is a rare complication.

VII.40 Likely symptoms of diabetic ketoacidosis include:

- **A** hyperventilation
- **B** extracellular dehydration
- **C** extracellular sodium loss
- **D** hyperdynamic circulation
- **E** coma.

VII.41 Complications of rheumatoid arthritis include;

- **A** anaemia
- **B** pericarditis
- **C** peripheral arteritis
- **D** jaundice
- **E** splenomegaly.

VII.42 Concerning acute gastro-intestinal haemorrhage:

- **A** the majority are due to duodenal ulcer
- **B** bleeding from gastric ulcers causes a higher mortality than from duodenal ulcers
- **C** any sedation is contra-indicated
- **D** the serum creatinine will be raised by absorption of blood from the gut
- **E** surgery is indicated when more than 4 units of blood have been given.

VII.43 Chronic diarrhoea is associated with:

A a Meckel's diverticulum
B carcinoid syndrome
C surgical truncal vagotomy
D diabetic autonomic neuropathy
E viral gastroenteritis.

VII.44 In a patient with sickle-cell disease, a crisis is precipitated by:

A suxamethonium
B hyperthermia
C acidosis
D halothane
E hypoxia.

VII.45 Dystrophia myotonica is associated with:

A thyroid adenomata
B the development of diabetes mellitus
C wasting of the sternomastoid muscles
D a high arched palate
E frontal baldness.

VII.46 The following can cause a spastic paraparesis:

A multiple sclerosis
B subacute combined degeneration of the cord
C anterior spinal artery thrombosis
D diabetic neuropathy
E syringomyelia.

VII.47 Drugs known to increase barrier pressure at the gastro-oesophageal junction include;

A prochlorperazine
B atropine
C glycopyrrolate
D fentanyl
E suxamethonium.

VII.48 Techniques that are suitable for use in patients with acute renal failure include:

A brachial plexus block
B lumbar extradural block
C spinal anaesthesia
D neuromuscular blockade with atracurium
E intermittent positive pressure ventilation with halothane.

VII.49 The following are true of acute pyelonephritis:

A the most common organism is *Strep. faecalis*
B the onset is usually sudden
C it is more common in women
D antibiotic treatment is continued until the urine is completely sterile
E fluids should be restricted initially to rest the kidneys.

VII.50 Alveolar hypoventilation is associated with:

A raised intracranial pressure
B emphysema
C pleural effusion
D asthma
E metabolic alkalosis.

VII.51 Likely causes of a large anterior mediastinal mass seen on routine chest radiograph include:

A thymic cyst
B lymphoma
C unfolded aorta
D retrosternal goitre
E diaphragmatic hernia.

VII.52 The following are true of asthma:

A the prognosis is the same no matter what the age of onset
B cromoglycate is of benefit in the acute attack
C the steroid of choice is methyl prednisolone
D IPPV is safe in the severe asthmatic and should be used to give the patient a good night's rest
E the patient should always be given humidified oxygen.

VII.53 Abdominal pain is a prominent feature of;

A staphylococcal food poisoning
B typhoid fever
C paralytic ileus
D lead poisoning
E Crohn's disease.

VII.54 Carcinoma of the large bowel;

A is more common in Europeans than in Africans
B will not have metastasized if it has not breached the serosal surface
C is more common in the sigmoid colon than the transverse colon
D not uncommonly presents with anaemia.
E is less likely to cause obstruction if in the ascending colon.

VII.55 Likely complications of abdominoperineal resection of the rectum include:

A deep venous thrombosis
B paralytic ileus
C air embolism
D post-operative atelectasis
E uraemia.

VII.56 Appropriate conservative measures in the treatment of hiatus hernia include:

A antacid therapy
B anticholinergic therapy
C weight loss
D histamine (H_2) receptor antagonist therapy
E steroid therapy.

VII.57 Acute peptic ulceration:

A commonly follows aspirin ingestion
B is frequently multiple
C usually causes perforation
D sometimes occurs in the duodenum shortly after severe burns
E is a complication of steroid therapy.

VII.58 Surgical hypophysectomy:

A is usually performed by an extracranial approach
B necessitates pre-operative steroid therapy
C may produce post-operative diabetes inspidus
D requires both mineralo- and glucocorticoid replacement
E is a contra-indication to induced hypotension.

VII.59 The following are true of osteoarthritis of the hip:

A the condition is virtually unknown in patients below 17 years of age
B pain is the prominent feature
C it is a self-limiting condition
D arthroplasty restores good function
E late sepsis is an uncommon complication of arthroplasty.

VII.60 Following elective hysterectomy, a 45-year-old patient is admitted to the intensive care unit cyanosed and with severe right-sided chest pain, sinus tachycardia and hypotension. Likely diagnoses include:

A myocardial infarction
B septicaemia
C pulmonary embolism
D bronchopneumonia
E spontaneous pneumothorax.

Paper VII Answers

VII.1 TTTTT

VII.2 FTTFF

A No — he should continue on propranolol up to the day of surgery.

D Not necessarily, unless hypertension and evidence of inadequate beta-adrenergic blockade are present.

E No reason, unless signs of cardiac failure are present, in which case propranolol may be contra-indicated.

VII.3 FFFTT

A Will result in rebound tachycardia and hypertension.

B Not necessary.

C Patient is probably already on this, which produces a vascular gland. Pre-operatively carbimazole should be stopped and potassium iodide commenced.

VII.4 FTFTT

A Stridor is a common presenting symptom.

C It is not contra-indicated, unless the airway is severely compromised.

E Parathyroid damage can occur during surgery.

VII.5 TTTTF

E 750 lb/sq in (51 atmospheres).

VII.6 TTFFF

C One should always monitor the temperature in a susceptible individual, but the condition is not always associated with hyperthermia and the diagnosis can be made from many of the other signs (rigidity, increased CO_2 output etc).

D Certainly not when anaesthetized.

E Dantrolene is the definitive treatment.

VII.7 FTFTF

A Vagolytic, not vagotonic.

B Not usually given orally, but it can be.

C Not, apart from problems with injections and small doses.

E Red herring.

VII.8 TFFFT

B,D Although in both cases nitrous oxide will diffuse in to the appropriate cavities, it would not produce sufficient increase in tension to create a problem. Anyway, you must have used it countless times yourself for large-bowel surgery!

C The leak may make it difficult to ventilate, but nitrous oxide will not affect the leak.

VII.9 TFFTF

B Is not directly related to hypoxia.

C Is treated by rapid recompression.

E The bubbles that do the damage are of nitrogen. Helium is less soluble, and helium/oxygen mixtures are less likely to precipitate the 'bends'.

VII.10 FTTFF

A,D,E Although these complications have been reported and, indeed, virtually anything can happen, the key word in the question is 'likely', and likely complications of the infraclavicular approach are **B,C**.

VII.11 TFTFF

B,E Respiratory depression produces a respiratory acidosis, but the drugs do not themselves produce a metabolic disturbance.

D Hyperpyrexia may occur.

VII.12 FTFFT

A Vasospasm often occurs post-operatively.

C Not so.

D Often better to have an awake patient to assess.

VII.13 TFFTF

B Halothane raises ICP by causing cerebral vasodilation.

C Phenytoin has no direct effect. It will lower ICP if the increase is secondary to fitting for which the drug was given.

E Classically described as raising it, although recent work suggests it may have no effect. It doesn't reduce it.

VII.14 TFTFF

B Anticholinergic only.

D,E Not antacids.

VII.15 FTFFF

A There is no impairment of gas exchange.

C Tachycardia.

D Not unless DIC intervenes.

E Not unless there is also abnormal placental attachment or inadequate contraction.

VII.16 TTTTT

All of these are true.

VII.17 FTFFF

Any diagnosis must fit all the (limited) information you are given. The history, temperature, leg held in flexion and pattern of bleeding suggest only **B** is likely.

VII.18 TFTFF

B Decreased due to vasoconstriction.
D Thiopentone produces peripheral vasodilation.
E Reduced in low output state.

VII.19 TTFTF

C Etorphine is licensed for animal use only (the safe answer is probably 'don't know').
E Indoramin is an alpha blocker — don't guess!

VII.20 TTFFF

C,E Both may precipitate an acute attack.
D Barbiturates are the classical contra-indication.

VII.21 TTTTF

D No time interval given; it takes some time for the sensitivity to occur.
E This is a red herring — there may be some obscure association, but it is not common!

VII.22 TFFTF

B This is for dead-space evaluation.
C Not useful, nor is it a standard test!
E The main problem is obstruction, not diffusion, and uptake of anaesthetic gases is not influenced by the transfer factor anyway.

VII.23 FTFFF

A Not essential; it depends upon the patient's condition.
C Artificial ventilation must be avoided until the bronchus is occluded.
D Not essential.
E Can be used, as cavity tension is not a problem.

VII.24 TTTTF

The anatomy of the larynx is difficult to visualize: try to find a three-dimensional model to study.

C,E This is the site for emergency puncture. The isthmus lies inferior to the cricoid cartilage, overlying the second to fourth tracheal rings.

VII.25 FTTFT

A Even bilateral phrenic blockade does not, in itself, cause respiratory paralysis; however, this is a unilateral block anyway.
D The risk of dural puncture is by interscalene approach.
E May follow a toxic dose of local anaesthetic anywhere by any route.

VII.26 FTTTF

A The basilic vein drains the ulnar dorsal venous network.
B It becomes anterior before it reaches the elbow.
E It perforates the deep fascia midway up the upper arm. Catheters are more likely to stick when traversing the cephalic vein where it perforates the clavipectoral fascia.

VII.27 FFFTF

A Contiguous means 'in direct connection with': it is not. However, only the parietal pleura separates the thoracic epidural space from the pleural cavity.

E There is not normally cerebrospinal fluid outside the dura.

VII.28 TFTFT

B Scalp to vertex, posterior to that is supplied by the occipital nerves via the cervical plexus.

D The anterior two-thirds of the tongue, but the whole of the mouth, gums and palate.

VII.29 TTTTF

B Via the greater superficial petrosal nerve.

D Bilateral innervation of the upper facial muscles.

E It traverses the interval auditory meatus. A branch, the chorda tympani, traverses the eardrum.

VII.30 TTTTT

Five parts of an MCQ = five nerves to be blocked for a successful ankle block!

VII.31 FTFFF

A Inability to synthesize bicarbonate results in metabolic acidosis.

C,D,E Not specifically with any of these: diabetes insipidus produces relative hypovolaemia, and hepatic coma produces metabolic acidosis.

VII.32 TTTFF

D Hyperaldosteronism will promote sodium retention and potassium loss.

E This will increase sodium retention.

VII.33 TTTTF

B Disopyramide is not a first-line drug.

D Although described in textbooks, eyeball pressure must be used with care: it can cause retinal detachment in myopics.

E Methoxamine is an alpha-adrenergic agonist.

VII.34 TFTFT

B,D Neither are associated with RBBB.

VII.35 TTTFF

A and **B** indicate the patient is taking digitalis; **C** indicates toxicity. **E**, unfortunately, is not true.

A Which just means a reduced heart rate.

D U-waves are a variant of normal.

VII.36 FFFTF

A Atropine is only suitable for ventricular ectopics occurring as escape beats.

B Propranolol may make ectopics worse.

C There is no reason to withhold higher concentrations of oxygen.

E Not suitable for multifocal ectopics that reflect myocardial ischaemia.

VII.37 TTTFF

A,B,C Stenotic or constrictive lesions tend to produce a fixed output state.

D,E Both can cause a low output state, but this is not necessarily fixed.

VII.38 FTFFT

A Not without further evaluation.
C Verapamil is reasonable treatment — but can precipitate asystole with beta-blockers.
D It may do, but it may indicate a problem on the right side of the heart.

VII.39 TFTTT

B The syndrome requires hepatic secondaries. The primary is usually quite small and the liver can metabolize any active substances released.

VII.40 TTTFT

D The circulation tends to be hypodynamic.

VII.41 TTTFT

E Felty's syndrome: splenomegaly, rheumatoid arthritis, leucopaenia.

VII.42 FTFFF

Note that the site of bleeding is not defined, it just says 'gastro-intestinal', and therefore covers both haematemesis and melaena.

A Not the majority of all GI bleeds.
D The urea, but not the creatinine, is raised by absorption of blood.
E We cannot give the indications here; read it in one of the standard texts.

VII.43 FTTTF

E Acute but not chronic diarrhoea.

VII.44 FFTFT

A Suxamethonium can cause many problems but does not precipitate sickle-cell crisis unless indirectly via hypoxia caused by failed intubation.

B Hypothermia.

D Halothane is not specifically a problem unless severe cardiorespiratory depression produces either profound hypotension or acidosis.

VII.45 TFTFT

B Not normally associated.

D This is a feature of Marfan's syndrome.

VII.46 TTFFT

A Especially in middle-aged women.

C Gives a flaccid paralysis of acute origin.

E Upper limb signs are much more obvious.

VII.47 TFFFT

B,C,D Anticholinergic drugs and opioids reduce the tone of the lower oesophageal sphincter and therefore reduce barrier pressure.

VII.48 TTTTT

D Atracurium is suitable because of its alternative route of metabolism, although this is pH-dependent, and so its action may be prolonged by severe metabolic acidosis.

VII.49 FTTFF

A *E. coli* is the commonest organism in acute pyelonephritis.
D Urine is NORMALLY completely sterile. Antibiotic treatment must be continued for longer than this.
E The patient must drink at least 3 litres daily.

VII.50 TTTTT

A Due to respiratory centre depression.
D Asthma causes hyperventilation initially, but in severe cases will eventually cause alveolar hypoventilation and pCO_2 will rise.
E Compensatory mechanism.

VII.51 TTFTF

C,E Neither produce an anterior mediastinal mass.

VII.52 FFFFT

A Prognosis is worse in maturity-onset asthma.
B Cromoglycate is of benefit in prophylaxis.
C Hydrocortisone is good enough.
D The incidence of barotrauma is high in the asthmatic.

VII.53 FFFTT

A *Staph.* is likely to produce vomiting alone.
B Pain is not a feature of typhoid.
C There may well be concurrent abdominal pain (e.g. post-operative ileus), but the pain is not a feature of the ileus.
E Pain may be masked by the bowel disturbances.

VII.54 TFTTT

B Less likely, perhaps, but cancer does not follow rules.
D Especially when in the caecum or the ascending colon.
E Because the faeces are less solid.

VII.55 TTFTF

C,E There is no particular reason why an AP resection should cause air embolism or uraemia, though a careless (or unlucky) surgeon could damage both ureters.

VII.56 TFTTF

B May be used in achalasia, but not usually in hiatus hernia.

E What would be the indication for steroids?

VII.57 TTFFT

C The vast majority are undiagnosed.

D Multiple stomach ulcers, not duodenal ulcers: though duodenal ulcers may occur later during recovery.

VII.58 TTTTF

E Elective hypotension is often used.

VII.59 FTFTT

A Osteoarthritis of the hip can occur in the younger age groups following injury or disease (e.g. Perthe's disease or a slipped femoral epiphysis).

C It is a degenerative 'wear-and-tear' condition that will continue to worsen.

VII.60 FFTTT

Note that there is no mention of how long it is since the operation.

A Not likely, especially with right-sided pain.

B Again, generalized septicaemia would not give the chest pain.

C,D If at about 10 days post-operatively, then **C** is the most likely, and **D** must also be considered.

E this is the most likely if shortly after operation.

Paper VIII Questions

VIII.1 Features of kyphoscoliosis likely to influence peri-operative anaesthetic management include:

A reduced vital capacity
B airway obstruction
C abnormal $\dot{V}/\dot{Q}$ ratio
D right heart failure
E hypocapnoea resulting from chronic hypoxia.

VIII.2 Likely causes of sudden death occurring under anaesthesia include:

A recent myocardial infarction
B aortic stenosis
C mitral incompetence
D second degree heart block
E ventriculoseptal defect.

VIII.3 Clinical features of APUD cell disorders which are of anaesthetic significance include:

A hypocalcaemia
B high glucocorticoid concentrations
C ketoacidosis
D anaemia
E depression of autonomic activity.

VIII.4 Appropriate anaesthetic techniques for microsurgery of the larynx include:

A a Pollard tube
B neuroleptanaesthesia
C apnoeic insufflation
D Sanders injector
E spontaneous ventilation.

VIII.5 Retro-orbital block:

A dilates the pupil
B causes enophthalmos
C reduces intra-ocular pressure
D prevents lacrimation
E increases the likelihood of vitreous prolapse.

VIII.6 End-tidal CO_2 concentrations during anaesthesia using artificial ventilation:

A are independent of fresh gas flow
B are usually measured with an ultraviolet analyser
C are independent of minute ventilation if CO_2 absorption is included in the circuit
D are elevated by opiates
E will rise steadily in a semi-closed circle system incorporating soda lime.

VIII.7 Inherited disorders likely to cause morbidity during anaesthesia include:

A malignant hyperpyrexia
B porphyria
C Pierre Robin syndrome
D Down's syndrome
E acromegaly.

VIII.8 Likely causes of post-operative confusion include:

A hypoglycaemia
B hypercarbia
C uraemia
D anaemia
E doxapram therapy.

VIII.9 The following occur in salicylate overdosage:

A coma
B acidosis
C haemolysis
D hypoprothrombinaemia
E hypofibrinogenaemia.

VIII.10 In the diagnosis of brain death:

A criteria cannot be tested in a spontaneously breathing patient
B caloric testing is used to test the integrity of the 5th cranial nerve
C serial 'flat' EEGs are required
D the absence of neuromuscular blockade should be confirmed with a peripheral nerve stimulator
E reflex movements of the legs may still occur.

VIII.11 The use of epidural anaesthesia for retropubic prostatectomy:

A prevents adequate assessment of blood loss
B is contra-indicated in patients over 65 years of age
C seldom causes hypotension
D contributes to fibrinolysis-related haemorrhage
E is contra-indicated in hypertensive patients.

VIII.12 Methods of reducing intracranial pressure prior to surgery include:

- **A** hyperventilation
- **B** sodium nitroprusside
- **C** spinal drainage
- **D** mannitol
- **E** propranolol.

VIII.13 Appropriate treatment for grand mal seizures occurring after surgical removal of a cortical meningioma includes:

- **A** intravenous phenytoin
- **B** thiopentone infusion
- **C** intravenous mannitol
- **D** intravenous clonazepam
- **E** hyperventilation.

VIII.14 Epidural analgesia in obstetric practice:

- **A** causes neonatal respiratory depression
- **B** controls blood pressure in pre-eclampsia
- **C** causes uterine relaxation
- **D** may cause retention of urine
- **E** may contribute to the effects of caval compression.

VIII.15 The following are likely to occur after amniotic fluid embolus:

- **A** cyanosis
- **B** hypofibrinogenaemia
- **C** hypertension
- **D** elevated central venous pressure
- **E** chest pain.

VIII.16 Concerning elective anaesthesia in neonates and children:

- **A** the normal tidal volume of a 4 kg infant is 20–25 ml
- **B** the ideal size of endotracheal tube in a 6-year-old child is likely to be 5 mm
- **C** the blood volume of a 4 kg infant is approximately 450 ml
- **D** the normal dose of neostigmine is 0.04–0.08 mg/kg
- **E** neonates tend to be sensitive to suxamethonium.

VIII.17 A 5-week-old baby boy of 4.1 kg presents with projectile vomiting and is booked for a pylomyotomy (Ramstedt's procedure). The following are true:

- **A** he is likely to be hypokalaemic
- **B** he is likely to be acidotic
- **C** the need for surgery is urgent
- **D** atropine 0.015 mg/kg is a reasonable premedication
- **E** awake intubation with a 3 mm plain oral endotracheal tube would be reasonable.

VIII.18 Halothane affects cardiovascular haemodynamics in the normocarbic patient by:

A a direct myocardial effect
B catecholamine release
C a direct effect on the sino-atrial node
D a peripheral vasodilatory effect
E vagal depression.

VIII.19 Ketamine:

A is a potent analgesic
B does not depress the cardiovascular system
C is rapidly metabolized in the liver
D maintains laryngeal reflexes
E may not be used in diabetics.

VIII.20 Appropriate premedication for a 12 kg child presenting for inguinal herniorraphy includes:

A 2 mg intramuscular morphine
B 0.1 ml oral nepenthe
C 36 mg oral trimeprazine
D 0.4 mg intramuscular atropine
E 500 mg rectal thiopentone.

VIII.21 Drugs that cause clinically significant release of histamine include:

A etomidate
B suxamethonium
C pancuronium
D fentanyl
E alcuronium.

VIII.22 Following reversal of a non-depolarizing muscle relaxant with neostigmine 2.5 mg and atropine 1.0 mg, a patient has difficulty in breathing, with tracheal tug, but is not cyanosed when breathing 35% oxygen. Correct treatment should include:

A giving a further dose of 2.5 mg neostigmine
B setting up a doxapram infusion
C testing the adequacy of neuromuscular transmission with a peripheral nerve stimulator
D administration of 100% oxygen
E respiratory stimulation with CO_2.

VIII.23 Suitable anaesthetic techniques for fibre-optic bronchoscopy include:

A spontaneous ventilation with nitrous oxide, oxygen and halothane
B apnoeic insufflation of oxygen and halothane
C local anaesthesia
D air entrainment using a Sanders injector
E emergence technique.

VIII.24 The following are true of these laryngeal muscles and movements:

A the posterior cricoarytenoids abduct the cords
B the lateral cricoarytenoids externally rotate the arytenoid cartilages
C the cricothyroid muscle tenses the cords
D there is no specific muscle that acts to relax the cords
E the cords are normally actively abducted in inspiration.

VIII.25 The following are true of block of the brachial plexus by the interscalene approach at C6:

A there is no risk of pneumothorax
B there is a risk of injecting into the vertebral artery
C the sheath lies between the anterior and middle scalene muscles
D there will be good relaxation of the shoulder
E there will be a unilateral Horner's syndrome.

VIII.26 The long saphenous vein:

A courses from the medial side of the foot to the femoral vein just below the inguinal ligament
B lies just behind the medial malleolus
C lies behind the saphenous nerve in the lower leg
D has many communications with the deep veins of the leg
E is superficial for most of its course.

VIII.27 The following are approximate equivalent levels for spinal segment and vertebral body:

A C8 and C7
B T6 and T4
C T12 and T9
D L5 and T12
E sacral and L1.

VIII.28 The trigeminal nerve:

- **A** emerges from the brain at the pons
- **B** divides beyond the sphenopalatine ganglion into its ophthalmic, maxillary and mandibular branches
- **C** supplies the lacrimal gland via the nasociliary branch of the ophthalmic division
- **D** supplies the sympathetic supply to the eye
- **E** does not supply orbicularis oculi.

VIII.29 The jugular foramen transmits:

- **A** the inferior petrosal sinus
- **B** the vagus nerve
- **C** the hypoglossal nerve
- **D** the spinal accessory nerve
- **E** the internal jugular vein.

VIII.30 The following statements about nerve supply are true:

- **A** the lateral popliteal nerve is more prone to damage than the medial popliteal
- **B** damage to the sciatic nerve is a complication of posterior fracture-dislocation of the hip
- **C** the pudendal nerve via the perineal nerve supplies the anal sphincter and perianal skin
- **D** sciatic nerve block necessitates the patient being turned laterally or prone
- **E** dorsiflexion of the great toe is from L4.

VIII.31 Acute hypokalaemia:

- **A** occurs in untreated hyperosmolar non-ketotic diabetic coma
- **B** precipitates digoxin toxicity
- **C** occurs following re-establishment of blood flow to a transplanted kidney
- **D** occurs during treatment of hyperglycaemia with glucose and insulin
- **E** follows therapy with carbonic anhydrase inhibitor.

VIII.32 The following are true of water intoxication due to overtransfusion with 5% dextrose:

- **A** epileptiform convulsions
- **B** muscle weakness
- **C** plasma sodium of about 140 mmol/l
- **D** urinary osmolality higher than plasma osmolality
- **E** treatment can include hypertonic saline.

VIII.33 ECG changes associated with intra-operative hyperkalaemia include:

A ventricular fibrillation
B high peaked T-waves
C low T-waves with U-waves
D ST segment depression
E ventricular extrasystoles.

VIII.34 Recognized effects of digitalis upon the electrocardiogram include:

A prolongation of the PR interval
B prolongation of the QT interval
C nodal rhythm
D ST depression
E tachycardia.

VIII.35 Elevation of jugular venous pressure is associated with:

A a Valsalva manoeuvre
B tricuspid stenosis
C sinus tachycardia
D constrictive pericarditis
E tricuspid incompetence.

VIII.36 A high venous pressure, hypotension and acute circulatory failure occur with:

A tension pneumothorax
B pulmonary embolism
C congestive cardiac failure
D venous air embolism
E haemorrhage.

VIII.37 Paroxysmal nocturnal dyspnoea is a symptom of:

A left ventricular failure
B bronchiectasis
C pulmonary stenosis
D ventricular septal defect
E aortic stenosis.

VIII.38 The following occur in primary myxoedema:

A bradycardia
B median nerve compression
C macrocytic anaemia
D flat T-waves on the ECG
E hypertension.

VIII.39 The following are found in hypoglycaemic coma:

- A moist tongue
- B low blood pressure
- C reduced tendon reflexes
- D hyperventilation
- E polyuria

VIII.40 Pre-operative pathological findings consistent with a diagnosis of phaeochromocytoma include:

- A decreased haematocrit
- B reduced plasma volume
- C decreased serum sodium
- D abnormal glucose tolerance test
- E increased excretion of homovanillic acid.

VIII.41 The following cause generalized pruritus with a rash:

- A mycosis fungoides
- B Hodgkin's disease
- C obstructive jaundice
- D pityriasis rosea
- E shingles (herpes zoster).

VIII.42 The following are likely diagnoses in a patient with jaundice and increased bilirubin in the urine:

- A infective hepatitis
- B obstruction of the bile ducts
- C liver disease caused by chlorpromazine
- D metastatic carcinoma in the liver
- E acute haemolysis.

VIII.43 Constipation resulting from reduced gastro-intestinal motility is associated with:

- A hyperkalaemia
- B hypothyroidism
- C hypocalcaemia
- D ganglion-blocking drugs
- E parenteral opiate therapy.

VIII.44 A 40-year-old female, admitted for elective hysterectomy, is found to have a haemoglobin of 8.2 g/dl and a reticulocyte count of 12%. This is compatible with a diagnosis of:

- A rheumatoid arthritis
- B chronic renal failure
- C menorrhagia
- D myxoedema
- E systemic lupus erythematosus.

VIII.45 In a patient with dystrophia myotonica:

- **A** spinal anaesthesia produces muscular relaxation
- **B** depolarizing neuromuscular blocking drugs exert their normal effect
- **C** non-depolarizing neuromuscular blocking drugs do not abolish myotonia
- **D** non-depolarizing neuromuscular blocking drugs produce an enhanced effect
- **E** diaphragmatic function is not affected by the disorder.

VIII.46 Flaccidity combined with extensor plantor responses occurs in:

- **A** motor neurone disease
- **B** the acute phase of poliomyelitis
- **C** the chronic phase of poliomyelitis
- **D** Guillain-Barré syndrome
- **E** syringomyelia.

VIII.47 Histamine (H_2) receptor antagonists have been shown to be of benefit in the treatment of:

- **A** uncomplicated duodenal ulcer
- **B** Zollinger-Ellison syndrome
- **C** Mendelson's syndrome
- **D** uncomplicated gastric ulcer
- **E** reflux oesophagitis.

VIII.48 A urine specific gravity of 1030 is seen in:

- **A** diabetes insipidus
- **B** impaired renal function
- **C** dehydration
- **D** diabetes mellitus
- **E** total parenteral nutrition.

VIII.49 The following are true of chronic pyelonephritis:

- **A** frequency and dysuria are the commonest presenting symptoms
- **B** there is massive proteinuria
- **C** pyrexia is rare
- **D** it is the commonest cause of death due to renal failure
- **E** it is a contra-indication to renal transplantation.

VIII.50 Alveolar hyperventilation is associated with:

- **A** hypoxia
- **B** respiratory acidosis
- **C** salicylate overdose
- **D** meningitis
- **E** hypertension.

VIII.51 Severe right-sided tracheal deviation is caused by:

- **A** right pneumothorax
- **B** nodular goitre
- **C** collapse of the left lung
- **D** left empyema
- **E** left pneumonectomy.

VIII.52 In chronic bronchitis:

- **A** spirometric changes occur early
- **B** clubbing is common
- **C** chest radiography is usually normal
- **D** steroids are usually ineffective
- **E** the likeliest pathogen to cause acute exacerbation is *H. influenzae.*

VIII.53 Classically the pain of:

- **A** a gastric ulcer is well-localized
- **B** hiatus hernia is well-localized
- **C** cholecystitis radiates to the praecordium
- **D** carcinoma of the stomach is worse after food
- **E** doudenal ulcer is relieved by vomiting.

VIII.54 Carcinoma of the pancreas:

- **A** is commoner in males than females
- **B** has a poor overall prognosis
- **C** is likely to present earlier if it is in the head of the pancreas
- **D** presents with diarrhoea
- **E** Whipple's operation is a curative procedure.

VIII.55 Ten days after a routine emergency appendectomy, a 19-year-old girl is unwell with a swinging pyrexia. The following are true:

- **A** an intravenous pyelogram should be done to exclude pyelonephritis
- **B** sub-phrenic abscess is a likely diagnosis
- **C** a pleural effusion would suggest a post-operative chest infection
- **D** she should have an urgent laparotomy
- **E** a high urinary white cell count does not necessarily indicate infection of the urinary tract.

VIII.56 Indications for surgical correction of a sliding hiatus hernia include:

- **A** anaemia
- **B** a tendency to bronchospasm
- **C** lung abscess
- **D** peptic stricture
- **E** associated pharyngeal pouch.

VIII.57 The following are true of chronic peptic ulceration:

- **A** it probably occurs in one in ten middle-aged men
- **B** a chronic duodenal ulcer never becomes malignant
- **C** chronic gastric ulcers commonly become malignant
- **D** most patients will eventually need surgery
- **E** pre-pyloric ulcers must be biopsied.

VIII.58 In a patient with a severe closed head injury:

- **A** intracranial pressure is dependent upon mean arterial blood pressure
- **B** intracranial pressure rises in direct proportion to the application of PEEP to the airway
- **C** fixed dilated pupils are always indicative of severe cerebral injury
- **D** treatment of choice includes hyperventilation to a $PaCO_2$ less than 3.0 kPa
- **E** leakage of CSF must be stopped immediately.

VIII.59 Common causes of haematuria include:

- **A** cystitis
- **B** hypernephroma
- **C** benign prostatic hypertrophy
- **D** tuberculosis
- **E** glomerulonephritis.

VIII.60 Recognition of malignant hyperthermia during anaesthesia is based upon:

- **A** failure of muscle relaxants to take effect
- **B** elevation of temperature above 39°C
- **C** severe metabolic acidosis
- **D** elevation of serum potassium concentration
- **E** ventilatory failure.

Paper VIII Answers

VIII.1 TFTTF

B Airway may be difficult, but it does not primarily affect peri-operative management.

E Hypercapnoea resulting from hypoventilation may influence management.

VIII.2 TTFFF

C,E Neither is associated with the occurrence of sudden death under anaesthesia.

D Only if it progresses to complete heart block.

VIII.3 TTTFF

Be careful to notice the words 'anaesthetic significance'.

D Not a feature of APUD cell tumours unless associated with haemorrhage.

E They are, if anything, associated with sympathetic overactivity.

VIII.4 TTTTT

C Insufflation with 100% oxygen into denitrogenated lungs. CO_2 builds up.

D Relies on the Venturi effect to deliver a reasonable tidal volume.

VIII.5 TFTFF

B It will cause exophthalmos.

D The lacrimal gland is supplied by the 5th cranial nerve from fibres originating in the 7th.

E It will reduce this by reducing intra-ocular pressure, and so to a certain extent options **C** and **E** are mutually exclusive.

VIII.6 FFFFF

A What happens to the $PetCO_2$ depends very much on the type of circuit: read about it.

B CO_2 is analysed with infra-red gas analysis.

C $PetCO_2$ is inversely proportional to alveolar ventilation by FRESH (i.e. CO_2-free) gas.

D The patient is being ventilated, so respiratory sensitivity to CO_2 doesn't matter: $PetCO_2$ may fall because of a reduction in metabolic rate.

E Not if the soda-lime is working efficiently.

VIII.7 TTTFF

D,E Although likely to cause morbidity during anaesthesia, neither is inherited.

VIII.8 TTTFT

A,B,C,E All are likely to cause post-operative confusion.

D Anaemia, unless accompanied by severe hypoxia, will not cause confusion per se.

VIII.9 TTFTF

A Mainly in children.

C Not a cause of haemolysis.

E No effect unless haemorrhage is catastrophic!

VIII.10 TFFTT

B 8th nerve.

C EEGs are not part of the diagnosis in the UK.

E True, due to spinal reflexes.

VIII.11 FFFTF

A Regional analgesia may alter blood loss, but doesn't prevent assessment.

B Epidural anaesthesia may be technically more difficult in the older patient, but there is no specific reason why it should be contra-indicated.

C Often, due to sympathetic block.

E Not contra-indicated, but one would have to be very cautious if the patient was not on treatment.

VIII.12 TFTTT

B SNP will increase the pressure within the closed cranium via vasodilation.

VIII.13 TTFTF

C Mannitol will reduce intracranial pressure, but will not suppress an epileptic focus.
E Not useful as a primary treatment.

VIII.14 FTFTT

A Local anaesthetics do not affect the fetus directly.
C Do not alter uterine tone.

VIII.15 TTFTT

C The shock is likely to produce hypo- rather than hypertension.

VIII.16 TFFTF

B A formula is (age/4) + 4.5, which gives 6 mm. The likeliest size is 5.5 to 6, though a small 6-year-old may need a 5.
C 85 ml/kg, i.e. 340 ml.
E Neonates are resistant to suxamethonium.

VIII.17 TFFTT

A,B He will have lost stomach acid and will have a hypochloraemic alkalosis with hypokalaemia.
C Surgery should wait until rehydration and correction of any electrolyte disturbance.
E Some paediatric anaesthetists do not like awake intubation of young babies.

VIII.18 TFTTF

B Halothane in a normocarbic patient is a sympathetic depressant.

E Vagal stimulation.

VIII.19 TTTFF

D Ketamine maintains the laryngeal reflexes better than other agents do, but will allow silent aspiration.

E No reason why, and if anything mildly elevates blood sugar due to catecholamine release.

VIII.20 TTTFT

B Aqueous extract of opiates: an unusual drug nowadays.

D A reasonable dose is 0.015 mg per kg to a maximum of 0.3 mg.

E Sounds a frighteningly large dose, but it is correct (40 mg/kg).

VIII.21 FTFFT

A,C,D Clinical probability, not pharmacological possibility.

VIII.22 TFTFF

B Doxapram is contra-indicated in patients who are partially reversed.

D The patient is not cyanosed on 35% oxygen: 100% O_2 implies more than a simple mask.

E Not a treatment of partial reversal.

VIII.23 TTTFT

Fibreoptic bronchoscopy is usually done under local anaesthesia and sedation.

D Only suitable for use with a rigid bronchoscope.

E The patient is made deep on halothane (or ether) and the bronchoscopy performed as the patient lightens.

VIII.24 TFTFT

B The lateral cricoarytenoids adduct by internally rotating the arytenoid cartilages.

D The thyroarytenoids relax the cords.

VIII.25 TTTTT

A C6 is above the pleura — but there will only be 'no risk' if you can identify C6 accurately

VIII.26 TFTTT

All these answers should be obvious to any anaesthetist who has kept his or her eyes open during surgery for varicose veins.

B It lies in front of the medial malleolus, an important site of venous access in fat infants and for cut-downs in severely shocked patients.

VIII.27 TTTTT

Either you know these or you don't.

VIII.28 TFFFT

- **B** Wrong ganglion: should be the trigeminal (gasserian), not sphenopalatine.
- **C** Yes, but via the lacrimal branch of the ophthalmic division.
- **D** Perhaps a bit of a trick: the SNS to the pupil (constrictor) is via the trigeminal, but there is also SNS supply via the internal carotid plexus from the superior cervical ganglion that subserves vasoconstriction.
- **E** Supplied by the facial nerve.

VIII.29 TTFTT

- **C** The hypoglossal nerve goes through the hypoglossal canal, above the occipital condyle.

VIII.30 TTFFT

- **C** The area is correct but via the inferior rectal nerve.
- **D** The sciatic can be blocked by an anterior approach in the upper thigh.
- **E** Useful when testing for the level of root lesions.

VIII.31 FTFTT

- **A** May occur as a result of treatment, but metabolic acidosis causes hyperkalaemia.
- **C** Hyperkalaemia will be reduced, but not excessively.

VIII.32 TTFFT

Plasma sodium will be very low, urine osmolarity will also be low with maximally dilute urine (SG=1.001).

- **E** Water restriction may be enough.

VIII.33 TTFFT

D Not associated with ischaemia.

VIII.34 TFTTF

B,E Digitalis shortens the QT interval and reduces the heart rate.

A common topic (see VII.35).

VIII.35 TTFTT

C Tachycardia will increase cardiac output and may lower venous pressure.

E Giant 'a' waves and cannon waves.

VIII.36 TTTFF

D,E Will cause acute circulatory failure and hypotension but not with a high CVP.

VIII.37 TFFTT

A,E PND is a feature of left-sided heart failure.

B Not a cardiac problem.

C Relative pulmonary hypovolaemia, not congestion.

D May occur if there is pulmonary congestion.

VIII.38 TTTTF

C Macrocytic anaemia is usually thought to be associated with the development of pernicious anaemia.

E Hypotension usually occurs.

VIII.39 TFFFF

B Stays normal.

C Brisk reflexes, perhaps extensor plantars.

D,E These are found in hyperglycaemic coma.

VIII.40 FTFTT

A,B These two are mutually exclusive — plasma volume is decreased and so haematocrit is likely to increase.

C Serum sodium is not greatly affected unless hyperglycaemia produces a diuresis, which is unlikely in view of reduced plasma volume.

VIII.41 TFFTF

You will not need to know much dermatology, but its relevance in general medicine can be important.

B,C Itch but no rash.

E No itch. The rash is not generalized except in the immunosuppressed.

VIII.42 TTTTF

It is important to learn the various permutations of what goes up and what goes down in jaundice of varying aetiologies.

A–D Any degree of obstruction will raise the urinary bilirubin. Chlorpromazine causes a cholestatic jaundice.

VIII.43 FTFTT

Two typically opposite answers.

A Hypo- rather than hyperkalaemia.

C Hyper- rather than hypocalcaemia.

VIII.44 TFTFT

D In myxoedema the haemoglobin would probably not be as low as 8 g/dl, and the reticulocyte count would not be raised.

VIII.45 FFTTF

A Only local anaesthetic directly injected into muscle produces relaxation.
E May be affected.

VIII.46 TFFFT

A The most common cause.
B,C,D Flaccidity only.
E Rarely — but there is no adverb of frequency in the question.

VIII.47 TTFTT

C They may help in the prevention, by decreasing gastric acid, but you are asked for help in the treatment.
D It is important that gastric carcinoma is excluded; the question says 'uncomplicated'.

VIII.48 FFTTT

A High urine volume of low SG.
B Inability to concentrate.

VIII.49 TFFTF

B Unlike in glomerulonephritis, protein loss is slight.
C Fever is the presenting symptom in one-fifth of cases.
E Obviously infection must be eradicated before transplantation, but renal failure caused by chronic pyelonephritis is not a contra-indication to transplantation.

VIII.50 TFTTF

B Respiratory alkalosis.
E Not with hypertension, but hypotension may cause hyperventilation.

VIII.51 FTFFF

The important word here is 'severe'.

A Mildly to right, but not severely.
C Moderately to left.
D,E Probably moderately to the left, unless the cavity is under tension, which is not stated.

VIII.52 FFTTT

A The usual spirometric tests (e.g. PEF, FEV_1/FVC) will not change until there is already a considerable degree of obstruction of the smallest airways.
B Clubbing is rare and should alert one to the possibility of bronchogenic carcinoma.
D It may be worth giving steroids a trial.

VIII.53 TTTFF

Not all patients show classical signs.

A,B Don't be tricked into thinking that because these options are worded the same they can't both be true: they are.
D There is not usually any definite relation to eating.
E 50% of patients with pain from gastric ulcer get relief from vomiting.

VIII.54 TTTTT

A True but only slightly.
C About 70% of cases are of the head; the earlier presentation is because it compresses the common bile duct.
D Diarrhoea is not the commonest presentation but is often a symptom.
E Unfortunately, it doesn't always work: for a peri-ampullary tumour the 5-year survival after surgery is perhaps better than 30%.

VIII.55 FTFFT

You are given only a very brief clinical summary: the correct answers must reflect that.

A There is nothing specific to suggest pyelonephritis.
B,C,E Swinging pyrexia suggests abscess: sub-phrenic or pelvic are likely sites. A pleural effusion would be further evidence for a sub-phrenic.
D The pus may be a wound infection — that would not require a laparotomy. Anyway, treatment is initially expectant.

VIII.56 TTTTF

A The implication is that the anaemia is secondary to bleeding from mucosa involved in the hernia.

B Bronchospasm increases the likelihood of aspiration, which is an aetiology of (**C**).

E Red herring — they occur at opposite ends of the oesophagus.

VIII.57 TTFFT

B 'Never' is uncommon in medicine. Nonetheless, chronic duodenal ulcers never become malignant (see Bailey & Love, 1981, Short practice of surgery, 18th Lewis, London).

C,E Malignant change is uncommon in a chronic ulcer. 20% of pre-pyloric ulcers are malignant — that does not imply that they were all benign initially.

VIII.58 TFFFF

B The cerebral compliance is altered so the intracranial pressure does rise, but not in a direct relationship.

C May be due to 3rd nerve palsy.

D Severe hyperventilation is not indicated.

E Not immediately.

VIII.59 TTTTT

There are other common causes of haematuria, and rare ones as well.

VIII.60 TTTTF

E Hyperventilation occurs in response to metabolic acidosis.

Paper IX Questions

IX.1 Following transection of the spinal cord above T5, factors likely to influence anaesthetic management of coincidental surgery within 1 month of the initial injury include:

- **A** hyperexcitability of autonomic reflexes
- **B** altered temperature regulation
- **C** contra-indication to the use of suxamethonium
- **D** exaggerated baroreceptor response to intubation
- **E** hypoglycaemia.

IX.2 A routine electrocardiogram on a 65-year-old man presenting for elective repair of a right inguinal hernia shows variable second-degree heart block. Appropriate anaesthetic management would include:

- **A** spinal anaesthesia
- **B** general anaesthesia with intermittent positive pressure ventilation and fentanyl
- **C** pre-operative insertion of a transvenous, fixed-rate pacemaker followed by spontaneous ventilation with halothane
- **D** inguinal field block
- **E** local infiltration during surgical repair.

IX.3 In the anaesthetic management of a patient with phaeochromocytoma, pre-operative treatment with phenoxybenzamine will:

- **A** reduce the severity of the symptoms
- **B** lower the blood pressure
- **C** decrease the haematocrit
- **D** prevent the hypertension caused by manipulation of the tumour
- **E** produce pre-operative sedation.

IX.4 An anaesthetic technique suitable for septoplasty should include the use of:

- **A** a throat pack
- **B** elective hypotension
- **C** nasal preparation with 10% cocaine
- **D** a non-kinking endotracheal tube
- **E** anticholinergic premedication.

IX.5 Intra-ocular pressure is lowered by:

A hypocapnoea
B halothane
C hypoxia
D morphine
E non-deplorizing neuromuscular blocking drugs.

IX.6 Which of the following statements are true of hyperbaric anaesthesia?

A working pressures with hyperbaric oxygen do not exceed 4 atmospheres
B hyperbaric oxygen therapy is indicated in carbon monoxide poisoning
C the partial pressure of nitrous oxide required to produce anaesthesia decreases with increase in barometric pressure
D rotameters are unreliable under hyperbaric conditions
E halothane is non-flammable below 6 atmospheres' pressure.

IX.7 In a patient with a hiatus hernia, anaesthetic complications at induction may be minimized by:

A induction of anaesthesia in the sitting position
B pre-operative antacid therapy
C pre-oxygenation
D topical anaesthesia of the larynx
E atropine premedication.

IX.8 Elective hyperventilation during anaesthesia for abdominal hysterectomy:

A reduces sympathetic tone
B increases the MAC for halothane
C decreases the cardiac output
D reduces the risk of deep venous thrombosis
E produces peripheral vasoconstriction.

IX.9 A 40-year-old man presents in the casualty department unconscious, breathing spontaneously with bilateral jerking movements of the limbs. Examination reveals papilloedema but no localizing signs, a PaO_2 of 11.7 kPa (88 mm Hg) and a pH of 7.14. Appropriate therapy includes:

A sodium bicarbonate 100 mmol intravenously
B intubation and elective ventilation
C emergency electroencephalography
D bilateral burr-hole exploration
E diagnostic lumbar puncture.

IX.10 If a patient, previously alert, remains comatose after successful cardiopulmonary resuscitation following ventricular fibrillation, treatment should include:

A hypothermia
B limitation of inspired oxygen concentration to 28%
C corticosteroid therapy
D doxapram
E mannitol.

IX.11 Acute paracetamol poisoning is characterized by:

A raised plasma alkaline phosphatase
B coma
C hyperventilation
D thrombocytopenia
E jaundice.

IX.12 In a child with raised intracranial pressure, scheduled for insertion of ventriculo-atrial shunt:

A induction is best achieved by the intravenous route
B neuromuscular blockade is contra-indicated
C fluid therapy should be restricted to 12 ml/kg/h
D the use of a cuffed endotracheal tube will minimize the risk of aspiration.
E cardiac dysrhythmias are frequently seen.

IX.13 In closed head injury, the following are contra-indicated:

A chlorpromazine
B clonazepam
C positive end-expiratory pressure
D elective intermittent positive pressure ventilation
E phenoperidine.

IX.14 A patient undergoing general anaesthesia for Caesarian section should have her trachea intubated:

A to ensure adequate fetal oxygenation before delivery
B to prevent regurgitation of gastric contents
C to prevent leakage of anaesthetic gases, thus ensuring rapid induction of anaesthesia
D in case amniotic fluid embolism occurs and bronchopulmonary lavage is required
E because of an increased incidence of tracheomalacia in pregnancy.

IX.15 The following are absolute contra-indications to epidural analgesia for an inguinal hernia repair:

A inadvertent dural puncture at the first space attempted
B ankylosing spondylitis
C multiple sclerosis
D allergy to local anaesthetics
E angina pectoris.

IX.16 Factors predisposing to the development of respiratory distress syndrome in neonates include:

A prematurity
B maternal diabetes
C maternal pre-eclampsia
D antepartum haemorrhage
E fetal congenital heart disease.

IX.17 Epidural opioids:

A are only effective in high doses
B induce respiratory depression
C produce itching
D are contra-indicated in thoracic surgery
E frequently produce hypotension.

IX.18 Immediate treatment of intra-arterial injection of thiopentone includes:

A intra-arterial heparin
B procaine
C phentolamine
D sympathetic blockade
E intra-arterial hyaluronidase.

IX.19 If an anaesthetic must be administered to a patient taking monoamine oxidase-inhibiting drugs:

A spinal or epidural analgesia is contra-indicated because of the abnormal response to vasopressors
B cardiovascular instability is likely to occur in about 60% of patients
C halothane should be avoided because of its action on the sympathetic nervous system
D local anaesthesia is contra-indicated
E premedication with droperidol is recommended.

IX.20 An abnormal response to suxamethonium can occur in patients suffering from:

A polyarteritis nodosa
B dermatomyositis
C systemic lupus erythematosus
D dystrophia myotonica
E hepatic failure.

IX.21 Concerning anaphylactic reactions to thiopentone:

- **A** the incidence is 1 in 5000–7500
- **B** a specific antibody has not been identified
- **C** they are more likely to occur in atopic individuals
- **D** they are associated with classical-pathway complement activation
- **E** IgE levels are unchanged.

IX.22 A 65-year-old man is admitted in acute respiratory failure. Results consistent with his condition being an acute exacerbation of underlying chronic obstructive airways disease with chronic bronchitis include:

- **A** a PaO_2 of 85 mmHg on 24% oxygen
- **B** a $PaCO_2$ of 65 mmHg
- **C** an actual bicarbonate of 22 mmol/l
- **D** a haemoglobin of 12.6 g/dl
- **E** a pH of 7.36.

IX.23 Adequate local anaesthesia for rigid bronchoscopy in a 70 kg man requires:

- **A** superior laryngeal nerve blockade
- **B** internal laryngeal nerve blockade
- **C** topical oral anaesthesia with amethocaine
- **D** at least 10 ml of 4% plain lignocaine
- **E** cricothyroid puncture.

IX.24 Considering the nerve supply to the larynx:

- **A** sensation above the cords is via the internal branch of the superior laryngeal
- **B** damage to the superior laryngeal will cause hoarseness
- **C** the internal branch of the superior laryngeal pierces the aryepiglottic folds
- **D** the left recurrent laryngeal nerve is the more readily damaged
- **E** the recurrent laryngeal nerves supply all the intrinsic muscles.

IX.25 The following segments supply the movements or muscles:

- **A** C5 and lateral rotation at the shoulder
- **B** C5–6 and flexion at the elbow
- **C** C6–7 supplies the long extensors and flexors of the wrist
- **D** C7–8 supplies pronation and supination of the forearm
- **E** T1 supplies all the intrinsic muscles of the hand via the ulnar nerve.

IX.26 The femoral vein:

- **A** is initially behind the artery
- **B** lies medial to the artery at the inguinal ligament
- **C** receives the long and short saphenous veins
- **D** is valveless above its junction with the long saphenous vein
- **E** becomes the external iliac vein behind the inguinal ligament.

IX.27 The following are true of the spinal cord:

- **A** the most important blood vessel (the anterior spinal) arises from the vertebral artery
- **B** the posterior spinal artery originates from the posterior inferior cerebellar arteries
- **C** the anterior spinal artery runs in the anterior median fissure
- **D** fine touch and position sense are carried uncrossed in the posterior columns
- **E** the thoracic and lumbar lateral grey contains sympathetic neurones.

IX.28 The ciliary ganglion:

- **A** lies at the apex of the orbit
- **B** must be blocked for cataract surgery under local anaesthetic
- **C** carries parasympathetic fibres from the oculomotor nerve that relay and form the short ciliary nerves
- **D** transmits sensory fibres, without relay, to the eyeball
- **E** does not carry fibres subserving lacrimation.

IX.29 The following are true of the vagus nerve and its branches:

- **A** it subserves sensation from the tympanic membrane
- **B** it subserves sensation from part of the external auditory meatus
- **C** the right recurrent laryngeal nerve hooks under the right subclavian artery
- **D** the left recurrent laryngeal nerve hooks under the left innominate artery
- **E** bilateral block at the base of the skull with a small volume of local anaesthetic gives good relief of the pain of mediastinitis.

IX.30 Division of the sciatic nerve at the level of the ischial tuberosity is followed by:

- **A** complete anaesthesia of the leg below the knee
- **B** loss of the ankle jerk
- **C** foot drop
- **D** paralysis of the hip adductors
- **E** paralysis of the rectus femoris.

IX.31 Specific inherited enzyme defects have been demonstrated in:

A phenylketonuria
B fibrocystic disease
C favism
D adrenal hyperplasia
E malignant hyperpyrexia.

IX.32 The following are minimum daily requirements in the adult male:

A 200 mmol sodium
B 80 mmol potassium
C 100 mg iron
D 350 mg magnesium
E 15 mg zinc.

IX.33 A profound bradycardia may be corrected by:

A applying pressure over the carotid sinus
B injecting a beta-adrenergic receptor blocking drug
C intravenous atropine
D intravenous isoprenaline
E eyeball pressure.

IX.34 Biochemical changes affecting the electrocardiogram include:

A hypokalaemia prolonging the PR interval
B hyperkalaemia depressing the ST segment
C hyperkalaemia producing high peaked R-waves
D hypocalcaemia prolonging the QT interval
E hypokalaemia producing tall U-waves.

IX.35 Causes of heart block include

A aortic stenosis
B atrial myxoma
C congenital
C syphilis
E amitriptyline therapy.

IX.36 An unchanged pulse rate occurring during and immediately after a Valsalva manoeuvre is found in:

A aortic incompetence
B Horner's syndrome
C autonomic blockade
D diabetes mellitus
E heart failure.

IX.37 Cardiac tamponade:

- A will occur if more than 120 ml of fluid accumulates in the pericardial sac
- B produces an increase in the central venous pressure accentuated in inspiration
- C results in a radial pulse of small volume that fades in inspiration
- D is unusual in viral pericarditis
- E is better treated with diuretics than by needle aspiration of the pericardial sac.

IX.38 In primary hyperparathyroidism:

- A serum calcium is increased
- B urinary calcium is decreased
- C alkaline phosphatase is raised
- D urinary phosphate excretion rises
- E rarefaction of bone is visible on chest radiography.

IX.39 Acute intermittent porphyria:

- A is associated with abdominal pain
- B is precipitated by barbiturates
- C is diagnosed by the observation of port-wine stained urine
- D occurs in West Indians
- E is associated with sickle-cell disease.

IX.40 Severe diarrhoea is a complication of:

- A diabetes mellitus
- B guanethidine therapy
- C hypercalcaemia
- D hyperthyroidism
- E carcinoid syndrome.

IX.41 Cramping pain of the lower limbs occurs in:

- A occlusive vascular disease
- B poliomyelitis
- C central prolapse of an intervertebral disc
- D thyrotoxicosis
- E hyperparathyroidism.

IX.42 The following statements, concerning the liver and its pathology, are true:

A jaundice due to monoamine oxidase inhibitors is cholestatic
B jaundice associated with halothane administration is more common in obese patients
C centrilobular hepatic necrosis is the classical histological picture seen in halothane hepatitis
D halothane maintains hepatic oxygenation better than ether
E pre-operative preparation of a jaundiced patient should include intravenous mannitol.

IX.43 The following are associated with ulcerative colitis:

A cirrhosis
B iritis
C psoriasis
D cholangitis
E arthritis.

IX.44 Sickle-cell trait:

A is found in subjects homozygous for the HbS gene
B presents as severe anaemia
C is inherited as a Mendelian dominant
D can be detected using the commercially available Sickledex® test
E is a contra-indication to the use of limb tourniquets.

IX.45 In a patient with progressive muscular dystrophy:

A tachycardia is a common clinical finding
B the myoneural junctions are not involved
C the myocardium may be involved
D thiopentone causes temporary peripheral paralysis
E inhalational anaesthetics are contra-indicated.

IX.46 Beta-adrenergic blockade:

A should be stopped two days prior to anaesthesia and surgery
B induces bronchospasm
C withdrawal may be associated with hypertension and myocardial ischaemia
D produces irreversible bradycardia
E is contra-indicated in conjunction with halothane.

IX.47 Complications of immunosuppressive therapy with steroids include:

A hepatotoxicity
B hypersensitivity
C diabetes mellitus
D osteoporosis
E bone marrow suppression.

IX.48 A metabolic alkalosis, persisting after elective partial gastrectomy despite adequate replacement of sodium chloride and water, is a strong indication of:

A potassium deficiency
B low serum calcium
C low serum magnesium
D water intoxication
E intracellular sodium depletion.

IX.49 A raised pCO_2 would be expected in:

A pulmonary embolus
B diabetic coma
C vomiting due to uraemia
D gross obesity
E chronic bronchitis.

IX.50 In a chronic bronchitic of the 'blue bloater' type:

A sputum is profuse and mucopurulent
B polycythaemia is uncommon
C arterial pCO_2 is normal
D cor pulmonale is a frequent occurrence
E alveolar gas transfer is normal.

IX.51 Factors predisposing to post-operative segmental lung collapse include:

A a recent upper respiratory tract infection
B cigarette smoking
C upper abdominal incision
D winter bronchitis
E healed pulmonary tuberculosis.

IX.52 In fibrosing alveolitis:

A the aetiology is frequently post-infective
B gas transfer is reduced
C hyperventilation occurs at rest
D the arterial pCO_2 is usually slightly raised
E chest radiography in severe cases shows pleural involvement.

IX.53 Primary treatment of extensive full-thickness burns should include:

A 20 ml fluid in the first 48 hours for each 1% surface area burned
B low molecular weight dextran
C transfusion of whole blood
D measurement of arterial blood gases
E steroids.

IX.54 The following would be of benefit in a proven gram-negative septicaemia:

A ticarcillin
B metronidazole
C cloxacillin
D gentamicin
E benzyl penicillin in large doses, given with probenecid.

IX.55 The following are true of herniae of the abdominal wall:

A a strangulated femoral hernia is an indication for urgent surgery
B a strangulated inguinal hernia is an indication for urgent surgery
C direct inguinal herniae are always acquired
D severe chronic bronchitis is a contra-indication to elective surgery
E incisional herniae occur early rather than late post-operatively.

IX.56 Factors associated with anastomotic breakdown following colonic surgery include:

A previous irradiation
B reversal of non-depolarizing neuromuscular blockade
C intra-operative hypotension
D steroid therapy
E anaemia.

IX.57 Following truncal vagotomy:

A gastric acid secretion is abolished
B megaloblastic anaemia slowly develops
C there will be gastric distension
D a proportion of patients will have diarrhoea
E late-dumping is more common than early-dumping

IX.58 A Colles fracture:

- **A** is a fracture of the lower end of the radius
- **B** results in backward and lateral displacement of the distal fragment
- **C** is particularly likely in elderly women
- **D** is usually greenstick in a child
- **E** is a cause of frozen shoulder.

IX.59 The following are true of carcinoma of the prostate gland:

- **A** it is less likely in men who have had resection of a benign enlargement
- **B** it is the commonest origin of bony metastases in men
- **C** skeletal metastases are radiologically denser than normal bone
- **D** hormone therapy helps symptoms arising both from the primary and secondaries
- **E** orchiectomy no longer has any role to play in the disease.

IX.60 The following occur in dystrophia myotonica:

- **A** testicular atrophy
- **B** frontal baldness
- **C** optic atrophy
- **D** ptosis
- **E** diabetes mellitus.

Paper IX Answers

IX.1 TTTFF

D If the lesion is above T5, the cardiac sympathetics are denervated and baroreceptor responses are not exaggerated.

E Not a problem.

IX.2 FFFFF

BEWARE — the primary problem is heart block and therefore the choice between local or general is of secondary importance.

C This is almost a right answer, but a demand pacemaker should be fitted.

IX.3 TTTFT

D Handling the tumour will release high levels of circulating catecholemines which will still produce hypertension.

IX.4 TFTTT

B Not necessary for a septoplasty, though it might be for an associated rhinoplasty.

IX.5 TTFTT

B Halothane reduces intra-ocular pressure by reducing blood pressure — unless CO_2 is allowed to rise.

C Hypoxia raises intra-ocular pressure.

IX.6 TTFFF

A The required concentration of N_2O is reduced, but not the partial pressure.

D They are not unreliable; rotameters can be calibrated under hyperbaric conditions. A rotameter calibrated normobarically will read incorrectly at increased pressure, but correction factors can be applied.

E Halothane is non-flammable below 4 atmospheres.

IX.7 TTFFF

C Pre-oxygenation is part of a 'crash' induction (rapid sequence intravenous induction) but does not minimize complications at induction, i.e. regurgitation.

D Topical laryngeal anaesthesia removes the protective cough reflex.

E Although intravenous atropine lowers barrier pressure, intramuscular premedication with atropine does not.

IX.8 TFTFF

B The pain threshold is raised with hypocapnoea so that the MAC is reduced.

D No evidence.

E Less vasodilation occurs, but not actual vasoconstriction.

IX.9 TFTFF

B Unnecessary at this stage and will mask neurological assessment.

D,E Both contra-indicated until the cause of raised intracranial pressure has been discovered.

IX.10 FFTFT

The implication is that the coma may be caused by cerebral oedema.

A Hypothermia was used at one time, but is no longer recommended.

B This may prolong coma!

D Doxapram is used as a respiratory stimulant. It is an analeptic, but analeptics do not reverse coma due to a cerebral insult.

E One would have to use mannitol with care if there was any risk of circulatory overload.

IX.11 TTFFT

C Hyperventilation only occurs late, secondary to hepatic failure.

D Paracetamol overdose does not produce acute bone marrow depression.

IX.12 TFFFF

B No reason why, ventilation allows pCO_2 to be controlled.

C Far too much, 2 ml/kg/h.

D Cuffed tubes are contra-indicated in children.

E Not frequently.

IX.13 FFTFF

A Often used to control hyperpyrexia.

B Anticonvulsant.

C Probably true, although it may be necessary to maintain oxygenation.

D Often used, though not now with extreme hyperventilation.

E A suitable sedative, although it masks pupillary signs.

IX.14 FFFFF

A Oxygenation can be accomplished perfectly well with a mask. An endotracheal tube does not ensure oxygenation anyway — what if the ventilator becomes disconnected?

B Prevents aspiration, but not regurgitation.

C Rubbish!

D Rare and therefore not an primary indication for intubation.

E Also rubbish!

IX.15 FFFTF

A Standard practice would be to try again at a different space, insert a catheter and leave an epidural infusion of Hartmann's in situ to try to prevent headache.
B Might be difficult, but not a contra-indication.
C It is impossible to prove that an epidural did NOT cause a relapse, but it is not an absolute contra-indication.
E This could generate much discussion — and for Part III this is just the sort of topic that you must be prepared to discuss.

IX.16 TTTTF

E Although it may be associated, it is not a prime predisposing factor.

IX.17 FTTFF

A Should be in low doses if effective locally rather than as a result of systemic absorption.
D Probably better than local anaesthetics, since they do not produce intercostal paralysis.
E Do not produce sympathetic blockade.

IX.18 TTTTF

E Not for intra-arterial injection, only for subcutaneous.

IX.19 TFFFF

B Probably fewer than 10% of patients show cardiovascular instability.
C Halothane is a sympathetic depressant.
D Local anaesthetics can be used, provided no vasoconstrictors are used.
E Not specifically recommended.

IX.20 TTTTT

A,B,C All are associated with liver dysfunction and so can cause problems, though rarely.

IX.21 FTTFF

A The incidence is more like 1 in 20 000.

D They appear to be an IgE-mediated phenomenon not involving complement.

E These are usually raised, although option **B** is still true at present.

IX.22 FTTFF

A This pO_2 is far too high for a patient who is in acute respiratory failure and breathing 24% oxygen.

D If the patient had chronic disease, he would be polycythaemic.

E The pH would be far lower than this — remember, this is an acute exacerbation of a chronic disease. His normal pH could well be 7.36 (a high bicarbonate compensating his raised pCO_2).

IX.23 TTTFF

D 400 mg plain lignocaine is a toxic dose.

E Not if the internal laryngeals are blocked in the piriform fossae.

IX.24 TTFTF

B,E The cricothyroid muscle is an intrinsic muscle, although it lies outside the framework. Hoarseness is caused by loss of tension.

C The internal branch pierces the thyrohyoid ligament and runs through the piriform fossa.

IX.25 TTTFF

D Pronation/supination is C6.

E T1 — true, but via the median nerve as well.

IX.26 TTFFT

C The short saphenous vein ends variably, but well distal to the femoral vein.

D There are valves more proximal: it is important to know if one needs to catheterize the femoral vein.

IX.27 TTTTT

A In a branch of this type remember that all facts (it is the most important, it is the anterior spinal, and its origin) have to be correct: here they all are.

IX.28 TTTTT

D Nasociliary branch of the ophthalmic division of the trigeminal.

E Secretomotor fibres follow a complex course from the facial nerve via the zygomatic branch of the maxillary division.

IX.29 TTTFF

D There is no innominate artery on the left: the left recurrent laryngeal nerve hooks under the aortic arch.

E Absolutely not!! Bilateral block would be exceedingly dangerous. Unilateral block of the glossopharyngeal nerve is sometimes used for glossopharygeal neuralgia, but there is inevitably spread to the other nearby nerves — look them up and work out what would happen with a bilateral block.

IX.30 FTTFF

A The saphenous nerve, a branch of the femoral nerve, supplies the skin down to the medial malleolus.

D Adductors are supplied by the obturator as well as the sciatic.

E Supplied by the femoral nerve.

IX.31 TFTTF

B Cystic fibrosis is transmitted as an autosomal recessive trait, suggesting an abnormal biochemical pathway, but not an enzyme defect.

E Malignant hyperpyrexia is a myotonic, not enzymatic, disorder.

IX.32 FTFTT

A 80 mmol sodium,

C 1 mg iron just replaces losses, but that needs an intake of 15 mg.

D,E Not figures that one tends to remember, but the problems of trace elements like zinc are becoming recognized increasingly in intensive therapy. Magnesium is an important intracellular cation.

IX.33 FFTTF

A This is a treatment for SVT.

B Beta-blockers would make this worse.

C By blocking the vagus.

E This is a (rather hazardous) method of vagal stimulation sometimes used to revert SVT.

IX.34 TFFTT

B Hypokalaemia depresses the ST segment.

C High peaked T, not R, waves.

IX.35 TFTTT

B Blocks blood flow, but is not associated with an electrical conductive block.

E May cause heart block, particularly in overdose.

IX.36 FFTTT

A Not unless aortic incompetence has precipitated cardiac failure.

B The cervical sympathetics are not involved.

C,D Autonomic blockade, or neuropathy caused by diabetes, will impair response.

E In heart failure there is a square wave change in blood pressure with no change in pulse rate.

IX.37 FFTTF

A Rate of development is more important, though probably upwards of 200 ml is needed to cause problems even if the effusion develops rapidly.
B CVP will be increased, but will still decrease on inspiration.
C So-called 'paradox' is an exaggeration of the normal. It is not pathognomonic of tamponade.
E Pericardiocentesis may be life-saving.

IX.38 TTTTT

A–E Parathormone specifically elevates serum calcium levels by mobilizing calcium from bone, and by increasing calcium reabsorption and phosphate excretion in the kidney.

IX.39 TTFFF

C Although the urine may change colour, the diagnosis depends upon chemical testing for porphobilinogen in the urine.
D Cape Dutch population in South Africa.
E No association except by coincidence.

IX.40 TTFTT

C Constipation if anything: diarrhoea causes hypocalcaemia because of malabsorption of calcium.

IX.41 TTFFF

A,C Intermittent claudication is a cramping pain; radicular pain is not.
D Not a feature.
E Hypoparathyroidism and hypocalcaemia cause cramping (tetany).

IX.42 FTFTT

A Cholestatic jaundice is associated with phenothiazines, chlorpropamide and others, whereas MAOIs cause a hypersensitivity-type of hepatitis (like halothane).

C Centrilobular necrosis is seen with chloroform: halothane produces a hepatitic picture.

IX.43 FFFFT

A Fatty degeneration and amyloidosis but not cirrhosis.

B,C Linked together with arthritis, but not with ulcerative colitis.

D Not associated.

IX.44 FFFTT

A Trait is the phenotype of the heterozygote genotype.

B Sickle-cell disease presents as anaemia.

C It is a Mendelian recessive.

IX.45 TTTFF

D Thiopentone is associated with exacerbation of familial periodic paralysis.

E Not contra-indicated, but must be used with care.

IX.46 FTTFF

A Continued up to surgery. This has been asked previously in the book.

D Can be reversed with direct-acting catecholamine infusions.

E No, though effect may be additive.

IX.47 FFTTF

A,B,E None of these are documented complications of steroid therapy, whether used for immunosuppression or not.

IX.48 TTTFF

A very difficult question to sort out — assuming that it asks for fluid and electrolyte disorders commonly associated with metabolic alkalosis.

A,B,C All occur as a result of metabolic alkalosis, particularly that caused by prolonged loss of gastric secretions.

D Unlikely if saline has been used.

E Possible but unlikely.

IX.49 FFFTT

A,C pCO_2 falls because of the associated hyperventilation.

C Although vomiting causes metabolic alkalosis, a uraemic patient would be acidotic and likely to have a low pCO_2.

IX.50 TFFTT

B Commonly polycythaemic.

C pCO_2 is raised.

IX.51 TTTFF

D It would depend upon the operative site and the state of the chronic chest disease.

E Not normally a cause of acute pulmonary problems in the absence of other causes.

IX.52 FTTFF

A There are many precipitating causes, of which a number are infective. More usually there is no known aetiology.

IX.53 FFFTF

A Far too little — fluid requirements are assessed six-hourly.

B,C Plasma is always used in preference initially. Dextran 40 should certainly not be used: dextran 70 is a reasonable substitute if there is no plasma available. Blood may be needed later.

E Not indicated unless there is direct burning of the respiratory tract.

IX.54 TFFTF

Ticarcillin (**A**) is a broad-spectrum penicillin — though most would probably use carbenicillin. Cloxacillin (**C**) and benzyl penicillin (**E**) are ineffective against gram-negative organisms.

IX.55 TTTFT

A,B The similarity of the wording is trying to suggest a distinction between the two types of hernia. There are some — but a strangulated hernia at any site needs emergency surgery.

D It may compromise healing, but better an elective repair (under local block, perhaps) than having to operate as an emergency (under general anaesthesia) when the hernia strangulates.

E They may PRESENT late, but they OCCUR early.

IX.56 TTTTT

Large bowel does not have as good a blood supply as small bowel, and conditions for healing are more rigorous.

B Neostigmine causes contraction of the bowel.

IX.57 FFTTF

A The 'cephalic phase' is abolished, but local hormones can still produce gastric acid.

B,E These follow gastrectomy, not vagotomy.

IX.58 TTTTT

- **C** Post-menopausal women have osteoporotic bones.
- **E** Patients must be encouraged to move the arm to prevent the joints becoming stiff.

IX.59 FTTTF

- **A** The two conditions tend to occur in different parts of the gland.
- **D,E** Orchiectomy is part of the available hormone therapy.

IX.60 TTFFF

- **C** Cataract, but not optic atrophy.
- **D** Not a diagnostic feature.
- **E** Not associated.

Paper X Questions

X.1 You are inducing anaesthesia with an intravenous agent through a plastic cannula connected to an infusion that flows freely. The patient suddenly complains of pain in that arm:

A if it is thiopentone, you must assume it is intra-arterial
B some agents have this side-effect; reassurance is probably all that is needed
C the patient may have suffered a myocardial infarct because of the hypotensive effect of the anaesthetic
D it is quite likely the patient will show evidence of local histamine release
E anaphylaxis is likely.

X.2 Likely causes of hypotension in the sitting position during anaesthesia for dental surgery include:

A emotional factors
B hypoxic gas mixture
C carotid sinus pressure
D vagal blockade
E increased baroreceptor discharge.

X.3 Suitable preparation of a maturity-onset diabetic, under treatment with an oral hypoglycaemic, presenting for repair of an inguinal hernia would be:

A setting up an intravenous infusion of 5% dextrose if the blood sugar was less than 4.4 mmol/l
B to delete the normal dose of oral hypoglycaemic on the morning of operation
C to administer the normal dose of oral hypoglycaemic on the morning of operation and give a single injection of 25 g dextrose immediately prior to anaesthesia
D to delete the morning dose of oral hypoglycaemic, but give 12 units of Actrapid® insulin intravenously prior to anaesthesia
E to give 24 units of Actrapid® insulin subcutaneously 30 minutes after the start of anaesthesia.

X.4 During anaesthesia for middle-ear surgery:

A moderate elective hypotension is advisable
B beta-adrenergic blocking agents should not be used
C air embolism is likely to occur
D nitrous oxide administration should be discontinued at least 30 minutes before application of the graft
E positive end-expiratory pressure is a suitable addition to arterial hypotension in reducing blood loss.

X.5 Intra-ocular pressure is raised by:

A hyperventilation
B hypoxia
C atropine premedication
D suxamethonium
E acetazolamide.

X.6 Suitable treatment for intense peripheral vasoconstriction includes:

A intravenous phentolamine
B sodium nitroprusside
C. propranolol
D dobutamine
E high spinal analgesia.

X.7 Blood loss during operation:

A can be regarded as minimal if the central venous pressure is above 2 mm Hg
B is accurately measured by weighing swabs
C is directly correlated with the haematocrit
D can be assessed by washing swabs and towels in water and measuring the haemoglobin concentration
E should not be replaced through a central venous line.

X.8 Factors predisposing to passive regurgitation include:

A suxamethonium fasciculations
B obesity
C head injury
D opiate premedication
E pre-operative metoclopramide.

X.9 Features of acute fat embolism include:

A unilateral tremor of the hand
B pyrexia
C carbon dioxide retention
D petechial haemorrhages
E retinal oedema.

X.10 During parenteral nutrition:

A sorbitol therapy may be associated with a lactic acidosis
B the normal daily potassium requirement is 15–30 mmol/day
C ethanol yields 7 calories per gram
D utilization of amino-acid solutions requires simultaneous administration of Intralipid® or dextrose
E more than 10% of the insulin given in an infusion is adsorbed onto the plastic.

X.11 High epidural anaesthesia to T1 impairs cardiac performance by:

A slowing the heart
B reducing venous return
C reducing sensitivity to endogenous adrenaline
D lowering serum cortisol response to stress
E reducing left ventricular end-diastolic pressure.

X.12 End-tidal CO_2 concentrations during neurosurgical anaesthesia:

A are an indication of the depth of anaesthesia
B rise as a result of air embolism
C should be maintained below 3.0 kPa
D measurement is inaccurate in spontaneously-breathing patients
E measurement is affected by the use of nitrous oxide.

X.13 Agents suitable for elective hypotension during surgery for an intracranial aneurysm include:

A sodium nitroprusside
B phenoxybenzamine
C trimethaphan
D isoflurane
E isosorbide dinitrate.

X.14 Suitable agents for the provision of pain relief in labour include:

A methoxyflurane
B enflurane
C bupivacaine
D trichloroethylene
E nitrous oxide.

X.15 Contra-indications to the use of spinal anaesthesia for vaginal delivery include:

A placenta praevia
B hypovolaemia
C breech presentation
D unengaged fetal head
E pre-eclampsia.

X.16 In a newborn infant suspected of having a tracheo-oesophageal fistula:

A the infant is likely to be cyanosed from birth
B saliva pouring from the mouth continuously is the cardinal sign
C a plain radiograph reveals total absence of air from the bowel
D barium contrast media are absolutely contra-indicated
E prophylactic antibiotics should be given.

X.17 Chronic deep pain:

- **A** is relieved by spinothalamic tractotomy
- **B** is characteristically made worse by transcutaneous nerve stimulation
- **C** can be relieved by mid-brain stimulation
- **D** is made worse by cutting peripheral nerves
- **E** indicates underlying organic pathology of the central nervous system.

X.18 Midazolam:

- **A** administration is contra-indicated in hepatic disease
- **B** hypersensitivity is complement-mediated
- **C** is a suitable agent for the sedation of patients with head injuries
- **D** is suitable for use in asthmatics
- **E** produces epileptiform changes on the EEG in susceptible individuals.

X.19 Adequate premedication with opiates:

- **A** reduces the amount of induction agent required
- **B** elevates plasma cortisol levels
- **C** suppresses beta-adrenergic activity
- **D** releases enkephalin antagonists in the mid-brain
- **E** may induce nausea and vomiting.

X.20 Drugs known to increase tone in the sphincter of Oddi during routine cholecystectomy include:

- **A** atropine
- **B** droperidol
- **C** morphine
- **D** glycopyrrolate
- **E** fentanyl.

X.21 Appropriate preventative measures in a patient thought to have suffered an anaphylactic reaction during a previous anaesthetic include:

- **A** antihistamine premedication
- **B** pre-operative disodium cromoglycate therapy
- **C** induction with etomidate
- **D** the avoidance of suxamethonium
- **E** complement stabilization with indomethacin.

X.22 A 30-year-old female is admitted following a suspected overdose of aspirin. An arterial blood sample taken before treatment, with the patient breathing air, is likely to show:

A a pH of 6.9
B a pCO_2 of 25 mm Hg
C a pO_2 of 76 mm Hg
D an actual bicarbonate of 10 mmol/l
E a base excess of −5 mmol/l.

X.23 Appropriate treatment for a supraventricular tachycardia occurring after pneumonectomy includes:

A intravenous propranolol
B carotid sinus massage
C intramuscular digoxin
D synchronized DC shock
E intravenous verapamil

X.24 At the level of the fourth thoracic vertebra, the following structures are related to the trachea:

A the aortic arch on the left
B the mediastinal pleura on the right
C the thoracic duct posteriorly on the left
D the right recurrent laryngeal nerve
E the right phrenic nerve.

X.25 Block of the brachial plexus by the axillary route:

A has no complications
B provides complete analgesia of the forearm
C is contra-indicated in sickle-cell disease
D will not allow manipulation of a dislocated shoulder
E occasionally misses the musculocutaneous nerve.

X.26 The following are true of the stellate ganglion:

A it is formed by the inferior cervical ganglion and the first thoracic ganglion
B it supplies sympathetic fibres to the head, neck and upper arm
C it can be blocked with 10 ml of 1% lignocaine at the level of the 6th or 7th cervical vertebrae
D block causes an ipsilateral Horner's syndrome
E during the block the patient should breathe slowly and deeply.

X.27 The following are true of the posterior primary rami in the thoracic and lumbar region:

A they all divide into medial and lateral branches
B they form plexuses to supply the backs of the upper arms and backs of the thighs
C the skin over the iliac crest is supplied by T12
D the lateral branches of L1–3 supply skin
E the lateral branches of L4–5 supply the skin up to but not including the skin that surrounds the anal margin.

X.28 The maxillary division of the trigeminal nerve:

A passes through the foramen rotundum
B passes through the pterygopalatine fossa
C receives the greater superficial petrosal nerve at the sphenopalatine ganglion
D can be blocked by an approach onto the lateral pterygoid plate
E has no motor components.

X.29 The lumbar plexus:

A forms within psoas major
B may receive a contribution from T12
C is normally L1 to L5
D supplies sensation to the whole of the anteromedial aspect of the thigh
E like the brachial plexus, is formed by the anterior primary rami.

X.30 In the neck:

A the internal jugular vein lies lateral to the common carotid artery
B the oesophagus is separated from the vertebrae by the prevertebral fascia
C the vagus nerves lie between the trachea and oesophagus
D the sympathetic chain is immediately posterior to the common carotid sheath
E the subclavian and internal jugular veins form the innominate (brachiocephalic) vein posterior to the sternoclavicular joint.

X.31 Situations likely to result in the development of acute hyperkalaemia include:

A rapid transfusion of stored blood
B adrenocortical insufficiency
C triamterene therapy
D tissue trauma
E anabolic hormone therapy.

X.32 The following concentrations, in plasma from venous blood, are compatible with which of the conditions. Na^+ 127 mmol/l, K^+ 6.0 mmol/l, Cl^- 85 mmol/l, HCO_3^- 18 mmol/l, urea 18 mmol/l:

A adrenocortical insufficiency
B hepatic failure
C renal failure
D carcinoma of the lung with inappropriate ADH secretion
E high small bowel obstruction with vomiting.

X.33 Likely causes of left bundle branch block include:

A ischaemic heart disease
B cardiomyopathy
C diabetes mellitus
D digitalis therapy
E mitral incompetence.

X.34 In a patient with acute myocardial infarction, the following sites of injury result in the following electrocardiographic changes:

A in anteroseptal infarction, ST elevation and T inversion in lead I
B in inferior infarction, ST elevation and T inversion in leads II, III and aVF
C in subendocardial infarction, ST depression in the chest leads overlying the affected muscle
D in anterolateral infarction, ST elevation in leads II, III and aVL
E in posterior infarction, ST elevation in lead I and aVR.

X.35 In the jugular venous pulse:

A the 'a' wave corresponds to atrial systole
B the 'y' descent follows opening of the AV valves
C giant 'a' waves are associated with pulmonary hypertension
D a large 'v' wave occurs in tricuspid incompetence
E cannon waves are associated with tricuspid stenosis.

X.36 A patient with infective endocarditis suddenly becomes dyspnoeic, with a blood pressure of 130/50. The venous pressure is raised, and systolic and diastolic murmurs become more pronounced. Likely diagnoses include:

A pulmonary embolism
B myocardial infarction
C prolapsed mitral valve cusp
D aortic valve rupture
E dissecting aortic aneurysm.

X.37 Functional consequences of moderately severe mitral stenosis include:

A decreased pulmonary compliance
B an increase in left atrial pressure
C hypercapnia at rest
D an increase in the left ventricular end-diastolic pressure
E a decrease in glomerular filtration rate.

X.38 Clinical features suggestive of the presence of a VIPoma include:

A hyperkalaemia
B steatorrhoea
C profuse watery diarrhoea
D hypercalcaemia
E acidosis.

X.39 The emergency treatment of myxoedema coma includes:

A intravenous hydrocortisone
B intravenous thyroxine
C intravenous saline
D oral liothyronine
E rapid warming.

X.40 Symptoms of hyperthyroidism likely to occur in a 25-year-old female patient include:

A reduced pulse pressure
B massive thyroid enlargement
C cold intolerance
D menorrhagia
E atrial fibrillation.

X.41 Causes of portal hypertension include:

A neonatal umbilical sepsis
B sarcoidosis
C Budd-Chiari syndrome
D anaemia
E oral contraceptive therapy.

X.42 Weight loss with a normal appetite occurs in:

A gastric carcinoma
B Addison's disease
C diabetes mellitus
D thyrotoxicosis
E tuberculosis.

X.43 Likely causes of a bleeding disorder which first becomes apparent during surgery include:

A acute fibrinogenaemia
B prothrombin deficiency
C plasminogen activation
D Von Willebrand's disease
E sickle-cell disease.

X.44 Massive transfusion of stored ACD (acid–citrate–dextrose) blood results in:

A a decrease in the plasma ionised calcium
B a metabolic, non-respiratory, acidosis
C hypothermia
D hyponatraemia
E hypokalaemia.

X.45 Petit mal epilepsy:

A commonly causes syncope
B is most common after puberty
C is precipitated by overbreathing
D usually leads to mental retardation
E has a characteristic EEG pattern.

X.46 The effects of noradrenaline are potentiated in:

A Horner's syndrome
B peripheral neuropathy
C treatment with debrisoquin
D treatment with guanethidine
E patients undergoing lumbar extradural anaesthesia.

X.47 Prednisolone:

A is used in the treatment of Addison's disease
B causes gastric ulceration
C causes hyperkalaemia
D produces osteoporosis
E causes hyponatraemia.

X.48 In the first three days after major abdominal surgery, examination of the urine shows a reduction in the excretion of:

A potassium
B sodium
C nitrogen
D water
E chloride.

X.49 Toxic effects of oxygen therapy include:

A corneal ulceration
B reduced pulmonary diffusing capacity
C retrolental fibroplasia
D convulsions
E pulmonary vasoconstriction.

X.50 In an emphysematous patient of the 'pink puffer' type:

A onset of dyspnoea occurs late in life
B alveolar gas transfer is reduced
C polycythaemia is common
D chest radiograph shows normal vascular markings
E cor pulmonale is a frequent occurrence.

X.51 A 57-year-old alcoholic is admitted to hospital with intermittent pyrexia, dyspnoea and copious sputum from which staphylococcus is cultured. A chest radiograph shows an opacity in the right middle zone with a fluid level. Appropriate treatment includes:

A diagnostic transpleural aspiration
B thoracotomy and lobectomy
C postural drainage
D drainage via an underwater seal
E intravenous antibiotics.

X.52 Signs of acute hypoxia include:

A muscular rigidity
B meiosis
C irregular respiration
D slow, bounding pulse
E extra-ocular muscle spasm.

X.53 The following occur in acute pancreatitis:

A retroperitoneal haemorrhage
B tetany
C pancreatic abscess
D pseudocyst formation
E hyperglycaemia.

X.54 The following are true of occlusive vascular disease of the large blood vessels of the legs:

A it occurs predominantly in cigarette smokers
B oral vasodilators are effective temporary treatment for intermittent claudication
C 50% of patients will eventually die of direct complications such as gangrene
D aorto-iliac reconstruction gives good results
E a claudication distance of less than 20 metres on the flat is an indication for urgent surgery.

X.55 Primary malignant tumours which commonly metastasize to bone include:

A uterine carcinoma
B rhabdomyosarcoma
C gastric carcinoma
D testicular teratoma
E prostatic carcinoma.

X.56 Indications for laparotomy following suspected abdominal injury include:

A tachycardia in the absence of hypotension
B left shoulder-tip pain
C abdominal distension in the absence of obvious signs of haemorrhage
D free gas under the right diaphragm
E bruising of the loin and dullness to percussion of the flanks.

X.57 At an outpatient appointment following gastrectomy for a benign ulcer, a 49-year-old man complains of dizziness that comes on an hour or two after meals. The following are true:

A the dizziness is likely to be relieved by food
B the dizziness is likely to be accompanied by nausea
C the patient should be investigated for insulinoma
D an anastomotic ulcer is likely
E he may be helped by taking a short-acting hypoglycaemic drug before meals.

X.58 In the first hour after a head injury, indications for operative intervention include:

A diminishing level of consciousness
B unilateral pupillary dilatation
C respiratory arrest
D CSF rhinorrhoea
E generalized convulsions.

X.59 The following are true of tumours of the testicle:

A trauma is a predisposing factor
B the most common presentation is enlargement of the gland
C most seminomas are radiosensitive
D gynaecomastia is a rare feature
E they may be part of the pluriglandular syndrome.

X.60 In a patient suspected of suffering from porphyria and about to undergo anaesthesia and surgery for acute appendicitis:

- **A** intravenous induction can safely be achieved with thiopentone
- **B** halothane is contra-indicated
- **C** serum sodium and potassium concentrations are low
- **D** blood urea may be raised
- **E** non-depolarizing neuromuscular blocking drugs should not be used.

Paper X Answers

X.1 **FTFTF**

It is not uncommon for patients to complain of pain or discomfort and then for local urticaria to appear.

C It says 'may', but this is scarcely a likely possibility—added to which the hypotensive effect of the thiopentone occurs after unconsciousness has occurred.

X.2 **TTTFF**

A Induction will then cause a reduction of the previously high sympathetic drive.

C Pressure during jaw support can cause inadvertent pressure on the carotid sinus.

D Vagal STIMULATION during surgery leads to bradycardia.

E Reduced activity produces hypotension.

X.3 **TTFFF**

C Oral hypoglycaemics must be withdrawn the day before operation; intravenous glucose will not cover for the prolonged effect of the oral drug.

D Just giving a single empirical dose of insulin without glucose is likely to produce hypoglycaemia.

E Treatment should be pre-operative, not intra-operative.

X.4 **TFFTF**

B These are often used as adjuvants in the hypotensive technique.

C Extremely unlikely unless the mastoids are involved.

D This is true if the graft is OVERlaid. It doesn't matter if the graft is UNDERlaid.

E PEEP is inappropriate: it may induce severe hypotension and the increase in venous pressure may make grafting more difficult.

X.5 FTFTF

A Hyperventilation (hypocapnoea) will lower it.

C Atropine does not affect intra-ocular pressure in the normal eye at normal premedicant dosage.

E This is an carbonic anhydrase inhibitor, which will reduce aqueous formation and therefore intra-ocular pressure.

X.6 TTFFF

Remember that you must be aware of the circulating volume before giving potent vasodilators.

C Beta-stimulants maybe, but not blockers.

D Positive inotropic agent only.

E It causes peripheral vasodilation, but is scarcely a suitable technique.

X.7 FTFTF

A Depends upon what other fluids have been given.

B,D Assume sucker bottles etc. have been taken into account.

C Haemoglobin concentration and PCV are both only a rough guide.

E It is better to avoid giving blood through a central line, but you may have to.

X.8 TTFFF

C,D Although both are associated with nausea and vomiting, they do not increase the risk of regurgitation.

E Metoclopramide increases barrier pressure and therefore reduces the risk of regurgitation.

X.9 FTTTF

A Not a characteristic feature, cerebral symptoms being mainly those of cerebral hypoxia.

C Due to severe impairment of pulmonary gas exchange.

E Fat may be seen in the retinal vessels, but oedema is not a characteristic.

X.10 TFTFT

B 40–60 mmol/24 hours.

D Utilization of amino-acids needs glucose: the balance should be 200 cal/g nitrogen.

X.11 TTFFF

C High epidural anaesthesia denervates the adrenals and therefore reduces adrenaline output, but does not have any effect on the myocardial sensitivity to catecholamines.

E LVEDP is a measure of ventricular performance: it is not affected by epidural anaesthesia in the normal myocardium.

X.12 FFFFT

A There are too many other variables for this to be reliable.

B Fall, due to reduced excretion.

C Below 4.0 kPa.

D No, the response time of an infra-red analyser is sufficient.

X.13 TFTFF

B This is a long-acting alpha-adrenergic blocker and is unsuitable for elective hypotension, which needs to be more readily controllable.

D Not really suitable for rapid control.

E Although this is a nitrate, the hypotension produced is minimal and insufficient for neurosurgery.

X.14 TFTTT

B Enflurane is not at present used as an analgesic, although it has been suggested that it may have some slight analgesic properties.

X.15 TTFTF

A Placenta praevia may be a contra-indication to vaginal delivery, let alone a spinal anaesthetic for the delivery.

C Regional anaesthesia is often used to allowed assisted delivery.

E This technique is indicated for the control of hypertension.

X.16 FTFTT

A Coughing and cyanosis will occur on feeding — contra-indicated once diagnosed. Delayed diagnosis may cause cyanosis because of aspiration (hence **E**).

C Air in the upper GI tract is a sign of the condition.

X.17 FFTTF

A Cordotomy of dorsal columns — spinothalamic tracts only carry cutaneous pain.
B May be helped.
E Any pain may have many causes, including psychological ones.

X.18 FFTTF

A Dose should be reduced, but is not contra-indicated.
B No evidence as yet, though it is unlikely because it is water soluble.
E Benzodiazepines are anti-convulsants.

X.19 TFFFT

B Certainly doesn't elevate them, and may prevent artificial elevation due to stress.
C No effect.
D Red herring — don't guess — why should antagonists be released?

X.20 FFTFT

A,B,D Anticholinergic drugs that will, if anything, reduce tone.
E Fentanyl probably does increase the tone. This is a rather contentious subject: we personally have not had any trouble using up to 5 μg/kg during cholecystectomy.

X.21 TTTTF

B This will stabilize mast cells and prevent histamine release.
C Probably the best agent to use under these circumstances.
E This is a red herring, although it sounds good!

X.22 FTFTF

A This would be unlikely initially; pH 7.1 perhaps.
B Respiratory compensation for a metabolic acidosis.
C The patient has normal lungs and is hyperventilating, so why should the pO_2 be so low?
E The base deficit (i.e. acidosis) would be much greater than this.

X.23 TTFTT

A,E Care must be taken if giving beta-blockers and calcium antagonists or the patient may develop intractable asystole.
C Digoxin is long-term treatment if the patient eventually needs digitalization: in the short-term, for what may be a short-lived problem, ouabain may be better.

X.24 TTFFF

C The thoracic duct lies too posteriorly and is not related to the trachea.
D The right recurrent laryngeal has already looped under the right subclavian artery: the left recurrent runs under the aortic arch and then up between the trachea and oesophagus.
E The phrenic nerves are more lateral.

X.25 FTFTT

A The axillary approach is certainly less hazardous than the more proximal approaches.
B,E Note that these are not mutually exclusive.
C A tourniquet is contra-indicated, but not the block itself.

X.26 TTTTF

A,B,C The anatomy of the sympathetic chain in this region is very variable; the stellate ganglion is only part of it. Block will extend from about C2 to T4.
E The patient should breathe quietly to help avoid pneumothorax.

X.27 TFTTF

B Plexuses are formed by the anterior primary rami.
E L4–5 do not supply skin.

X.28 TTTTT

C From the facial, eventually secretomotor to the lacrimal gland.
D Lies anterosuperior in this approach.
E Not in the true sense, though it carries secretomotor (C).

X.29 TTFTT

C Normally L1 to L4.
D T12 supplies the skin over the lateral buttock (subcostal nerve) and iliac crest (posterior primary ramus) but that is not 'anteromedial'.

X.30 TTFTT

C The recurrent laryngeal nerves, not the vagi, lie between the trachea and oesophagus.

X.31 TTTTF

A The potassium is rapidly re-taken up by the red cells.
B Low sodium, high potassium.
C A potassium-conserving diuretic which can cause hyperkalaemia if used inadvisedly.
E Red herring.

X.32 TFTFF

In a question giving laboratory findings, identify the abnormalities and attempt a provisional diagnosis before looking at the branches.

B Urea is low in hepatic failure.
D Urea low.
E Unlikely to be acidotic, and would be hypokalaemic if anything.

X.33 TTFFF

C Ischaemic heart disease is more likely in diabetics, but diabetes per se is not associated with bundle branch block.
D Digitalis can cause almost any type of dysrhythmia, but not LBBB.
E Aortic but not mitral valve disease.

X.34 TTTFF

D Elevation in lead I, aVL and V4–6.
E This would be anteroseptal. Posterior infarction is difficult: there are likely to be tall R-waves in V1–2.

X.35 TTTTF

A Elevated atrial systolic pressure.
D Abnormal venous filling.
E Tricuspid incompetence, not stenosis.

X.36 FFTTF

A,B,E Will not explain the systolic and diastolic murmurs.
C,D The valve lesion is more likely to be aortic than mitral in view of the low diastolic pressure, although mitral valve destruction is probably more likely to cause the pulmonary symptoms and cardiac failure.

X.37 TTFFF

Many of the physical signs of mitral stenosis are demonstrable before the condition has progressed enough to cause symptoms.

- **C** Hypercapnia implies hypoventilation or reduced drive to ventilation.
- **D** The LV is beyond the stenosed valve, and so LVEDP will not be affected.
- **E** GFR may be reduced if the stenosis is severe enough to cause heart failure.

X.38 FFTTT

VIPomas produce 'vasoactive intestinal peptide' and probably other active substances as well.

- **A** Hypokalaemia, if anything, as a result of the associated diarrhoea.
- **B** Not associated with vipomas.

X.39 TFFTF

- **B** Intravenous T3, but not thyroxine.
- **C** Beware salt overload.
- **E** Slow rewarming.

X.40 FTTFF

- **A** Hyperdynamic circulation will increase pulse pressure.
- **D** Amenorrhoea is more likely.
- **E** Atrial fibrillation is common in the older patient with thyrotoxicosis, but not in a 25-year-old.

X.41 TTTFT

- **D** Produces a hyperdynamic systemic circulation, but not portal hypertension.

X.42 TFTTTF

- **B,E** Both conditions cause poor appetite, debility and weight loss.

X.43 TTTTF

E Sickle-cell disease causes problems because of the formation of peripheral micro-emboli, but it is not a bleeding disorder.

X.44 TTTFF

A The citrate combines with Ca^{2+}.

E Hyperkalaemia if anything, although the potassium is re-taken up by the red cells fairly quickly once warmed up within the circulation.

X.45 FFFFT

A Patients go momentarily blank but do not usually fall down.

B It is commoner before puberty and tends to regress in later life.

C Overbreathing causes hypocapnia, and that is a cause of cerebral irritability that can precipitate epileptiform convulsions in susceptible patients. Petit mal has a different mechanism.

D Not necessarily.

X.46 FFFFF

A Results from cervical sympathetic block.

B,E Both affect peripheral vasodilation, which may be reversed by noradrenaline, but not abnormally so.

C,D Reduced due to impaired release of noradrenaline.

X.47 TTFTF

C,E Steroid therapy causes hypokalaemia and sodium retention.

X.48 FTFTT

A Potassium losses are increased following the trauma of operation.

C Nitrogen losses are increased by catabolism and there is negative nitrogen balance.

X.49 FTTTT

A Only a complication of direct application of gas to the eyes.

D Fits can occur at partial pressures of oxygen above 2 atmospheres, so this is 'true' because the question does not specify normal atmospheric pressure.

X.50 TTFFF

C Relatively uncommon, unlike the 'blue bloater'.

D Vessels are attenuated.

E Infrequent, but when it occurs it is usually terminal.

X.51 TFTFT

A Assuming that this is an abscess cavity with a fluid level, diagnostic aspiration would be helpful.

B Not unless conservative treatment fails.

D Not unless there is an associated bronchopleural fistula.

X.52 TFTTT

B Mydriasis rather than meiosis.

D The question implies simple acute primary hypoxia, rather than respiratory failure with a high pCO_2 (which would be likely to cause a tachycardia).

X.53 TTTTT

X.54 TFFTF

B Vasodilators aid skin blood flow and can help trophic ulcers to heal, but they do not improve muscle blood flow.

C Cardiac and cerebral complications of arteriosclerosis kill most patients.

E If the patient does not want or need to walk that distance, then there is no need for operation.

X.55 FTTFT

Note inclusion of the word 'commonly'.

A Localized and transperitoneal spread.

D Intra-abdominal spread.

X.56 FTFTF

A Analgesia should be the first-line treatment.

C This may be due to toxic gastric distension or paralytic ileus.

E Retroperitoneal haematomas are not necessarily an indication for operation.

X.57 TTFFF

The patient is likely to be suffering from late-dumping syndrome, which is caused by hypoglycaemia.

C Rare and often missed — but there is no particular reason to suspect one here.

D Not a symptom of recurrent ulcer.

E Hypoglycaemic drugs may help in early-dumping.

X.58 TTFFF

C Respiratory arrest may be because of brain-stem contusion or cerebral oedema: neither are indications for operation.

D Not an indication for immediate operation.

E A possible indication for anticonvulsant therapy, but not for operation.

X.59 FTTTF

A Trauma may draw the patient's attention to the swelling, and undescended testes (which are more liable to trauma) are more likely to become malignant. Trauma is not of itself a factor.

X.60 FFTTF

- **A** Barbiturates are contra-indicated — and you should certainly know *that* by now!
- **B** No, it may be used.
- **C,D** These biochemical findings can be present in porphyria.
- **E** Are not associated with exacerbations and have been reported as safe.

Index

Questions are listed under broad headings only. There is some overlap between categories; no questions are listed more than once. Roman numerals indicate the number of the paper, and the arabic number that follows is the number of the question on the paper.

Anaesthesia

Anatomy